# Advanced Strategies for Tooth Extraction in Dentistry

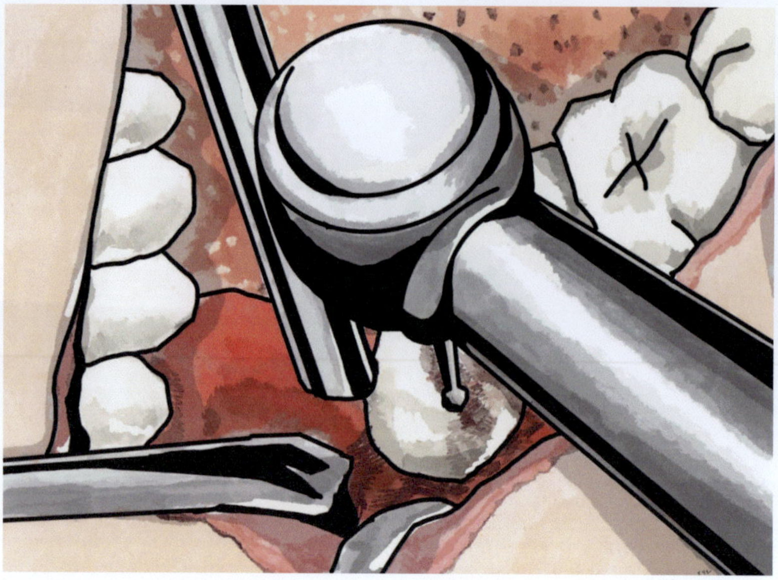

(Jee Ho Lee, DDS, PhD)

Seong-Gon Kim • Ji-Hyeon Oh
Dae-Seok Hwang

# Advanced Strategies for Tooth Extraction in Dentistry

## Beyond Basics

Springer

Seong-Gon Kim
Oral and Maxillofacial Surgery
Gangneung–Wonju National University
Gangneung, Gangwon-do
Korea (Republic of)

Ji-Hyeon Oh
Oral and Maxillofacial Surgery
Gangneung–Wonju National University
Gangneung, Gangwon-do
Korea (Republic of)

Dae-Seok Hwang
Oral and Maxillofacial Surgery
Pusan National University
Dental School
Yangsan
Gyeongsangnam-do
Korea (Republic of)

ISBN 978-981-97-6534-8 ISBN 978-981-97-6532-4 (eBook)
https://doi.org/10.1007/978-981-97-6532-4



This Springer imprint is published by the registered company Springer Nature Singapore Pte Ltd.
The registered company address is: 152 Beach Road, #21-01/04 Gateway East, Singapore 189721, Singapore

# Preface

Tooth extraction, a procedure frequently practiced by dentists, is often covered as a subsection in oral and maxillofacial surgery textbooks. While some atlases provide detailed, step-by-step guides to tooth extraction, these resources, though valuable for beginners, may not fully address the complexities encountered in daily practice. The reality is that tooth extraction can be complicated by a patient's unique conditions, emphasizing the need to consider the tooth not just as an isolated entity, but as a part of the body influenced by overall health. Understanding a patient's systemic condition is crucial for a smooth and uneventful procedure.

Recognizing these challenges, *Advanced Strategies for Tooth Extraction in Dentistry: Beyond Basics* has been meticulously crafted to cater to the nuanced needs of dental students, trainees, and examinees. This book goes beyond the basics, aligning with dental curricula and examination requirements, and focuses on imparting the knowledge and skills necessary for advanced tooth extraction procedures. It provides comprehensive coverage of the subject, preparing readers to navigate the challenges of their dental education and examinations effectively.

Each chapter in *Advanced Strategies for Tooth Extraction in Dentistry* is systematically structured, concentrating on essential areas frequently included in dental curricula and examinations. The content is presented clearly and concisely, facilitating efficient learning and a deep understanding of advanced tooth extraction techniques. Case examples and clinical scenarios are integrated throughout the book, bridging theory with practical application. These scenarios not only reinforce learning but also simulate the types of questions that appear in dental examinations, offering valuable practice and insight into examination techniques.

A cornerstone of this book is its commitment to evidence-based principles. *Advanced Strategies for Tooth Extraction in Dentistry* is up-to-date with the latest advancements in oral and maxillofacial surgery, ensuring the content adheres to both academic and clinical standards in dental education. Readers can trust that the strategies and practices presented are rooted in rigorous research and reflect the highest standards of patient care.

In conclusion, *Advanced Strategies for Tooth Extraction in Dentistry: Beyond Basics* is an invaluable resource that enhances the learning experience for dental students, trainees, and examinees. It not only addresses the educational and examination needs of dental professionals but also serves as an indispensable guide for their success in the demanding field of dentistry.

We wish to extend our heartfelt gratitude to our families and colleagues. Their unwavering support and contributions were instrumental in the completion of this work. Without them, this book would not have been possible.

Gangneung, Gangwon-do, Republic of Korea Seong-Gon Kim
Gangneung, Gangwon-do, Republic of Korea Ji-Hyeon Oh
Yangsan, Gyeongsangnam-do, Republic of Korea Dae-Seok Hwang

# Contents

## About the Authors

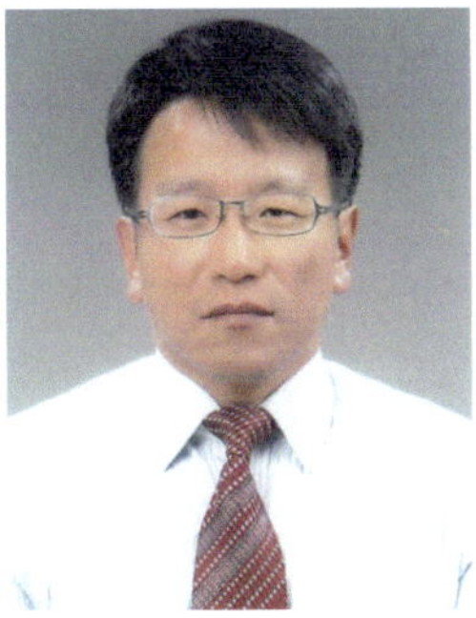

**Seong-Gon Kim, D.D.S., Ph.D.,** is a distinguished Professor at the Department of Oral and Maxillofacial Surgery, School of Dentistry, Gangneung-Wonju National University, Republic of Korea. With a dental degree and Ph.D. from Seoul National University, Dr. Kim has forged an illustrious career, marked by significant academic and professional achievements. His expertise is rooted in oral pathology, and he has held various esteemed positions, including a Fellowship at Seoul National University Hospital and an instructor role at Hallym University.

Dr. Kim's scholarly contributions are substantial, having authored numerous influential publications in international journals. His research spans a wide range of topics in oral and maxillofacial surgery, demonstrating his commitment to advancing the field. As an Editor-in-Chief and a member of various editorial committees, he has significantly influenced academic discourse. His dedication to his field is further exemplified by his role as Vice President of the Korean Society of Sericultural Science since 2021.

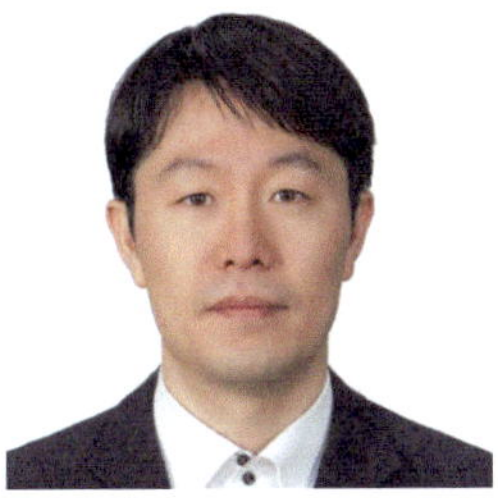

**Dae-Seok Hwang, D.D.S., Ph.D.,** is a distinguished Professor at the Department of Oral and Maxillofacial Surgery, School of Dentistry, Pusan National University, Republic of Korea. With a dental degree and Ph.D. from Pusan National University, Dr. Hwang has forged an illustrious career, marked by significant academic and professional achievements. His expertise is rooted in Oral and Maxillofacial Surgery, and he has held various esteemed positions, including a Fellowship and instructor at Pusan National University Hospital.

Dr. Hwang's scholarly contributions are substantial, having authored numerous influential publications in international journals. His research spans a wide range of topics in oral and maxillofacial surgery, demonstrating his commitment to advancing the field. As an Editor of *Maxillofacial Plastic and Reconstructive Surgery* (MPRS) and a member of various editorial committees, he has significantly influenced academic discourse.

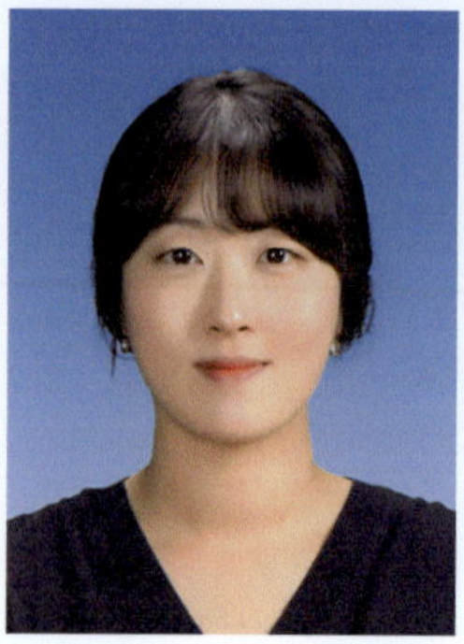

**Ji-Hyeon Oh, D.D.S., Ph.D.,** is a distinguished oral and maxillofacial surgeon, bringing a wealth of knowledge and expertise to the field. Dr. Oh graduated with a D.D.S. from the College of Dentistry at Yonsei University, Republic of Korea, and continued to pursue academic excellence by earning a Ph.D. from the Graduate School of Yonsei University, Republic of Korea. Dr. Oh has built a robust career in oral and maxillofacial surgery, demonstrating a commitment to both education and clinical practice.

Dr. Oh served as a Fellow in the Department of Oral and Maxillofacial Surgery at Gangneung-Wonju National University's Dental Hospital, Republic of Korea, followed by roles as a Clinical Assistant Professor in the same department. Currently, Dr. Oh holds the position of Assistant Professor in the Department of Oral and Maxillofacial Surgery at Gangneung-Wonju National University, Republic of Korea, contributing her expertise to the academic and clinical aspects.

# 1 Introduction to Advanced Tooth Extraction: Surgical Principle

## Contents



## 1.1 Introduction

Welcome to the pioneering realm of advanced tooth extraction, an essential surgical procedure that every dental practitioner must master. This book chapter, being the first stepping stone in your journey, strives to offer comprehensive knowledge, strategies, and insights into modern tooth extraction principles, including the incision, suturing, dressing, and closing remarks. Whether you are a dental student just beginning to explore this technique or an experienced dentist seeking to update your skills, this resource is designed to serve as a practical guide to complex tooth extractions, catering to a broad spectrum of learners.

Tooth extraction, at its core, is an integral part of dentistry. Despite advancements in oral healthcare and preventative measures, there are instances where a tooth cannot be saved and must



S.-G. Kim et al., *Advanced Strategies for Tooth Extraction in Dentistry*,
https://doi.org/10.1007/978-981-97-6532-4_1

be removed. This could be due to severe decay, periodontal disease, orthodontic correction, impaction, or even trauma. Over the years, the procedure has evolved significantly, with advanced techniques that aim to make the extraction process less invasive and more comfortable for patients, while ensuring rapid recovery.

However, the art and science of tooth extraction encompass more than just the physical removal of the tooth. It demands a thorough understanding of dental anatomy, excellent clinical judgment, precise surgical skills, and the ability to manage potential complications. In essence, it requires a delicate blend of knowledge and practice to achieve mastery.

This chapter begins by introducing the fundamental surgical principle behind advanced tooth extraction. This encompasses understanding the rationale for tooth extraction, evaluating patient factors, and the fundamental principle of "atraumatic" extraction, which strives to preserve the surrounding tissue structures as much as possible during the procedure. In subsequent sections, we will systematically explore incision techniques, suturing strategies, and dressing, each critical in their roles for a successful tooth extraction.

The purpose of this chapter is to equip you with the fundamental surgical principles and technical skills, thereby enabling you to perform tooth extractions with greater confidence, precision, and care. In doing so, we hope to contribute to your journey in becoming not only a proficient dentist but also a compassionate caregiver. Your journey toward mastering advanced tooth extraction begins here, and we trust it will be an enlightening and rewarding one.

## 1.2 Incision

In any surgical procedure, the incision serves as the opening note, setting the tone for the rest of the operation. As it pertains to tooth extraction, a well-planned and precisely executed incision is critical in maintaining the integrity of the surrounding tissue and facilitating subsequent steps of the extraction process [1].

### 1.2.1 The Principle of Incision

Incisions in dental surgeries are designed with two primary objectives: to provide adequate access to the surgical site and to preserve the function and aesthetics of the oral structures as much as possible. The approach, direction, and depth of an incision, therefore, must be meticulously planned in accordance with these principles. Basic principles can be enlisted as follows:

1. The size and direction of the incision should be parallel to the minimal tension line.
2. The incision should be made at a consistent depth to the full thickness of the skin in one stroke.
3. When using the blade, start at a right angle initially, diagonal in the middle, and finish at a right angle (Fig. 1.1).
4. Generally, incisions are made at a right angle to the skin surface, but modified incisions first make a right-angle cut, then after separating, slightly remove the inner side of the incision margin at an angle with scissors. This means that even if tension is applied after suturing, the wound site does not strain, resulting in fewer scars.
5. If possible, avoid hair follicles, blood vessels, nerves, etc., during the incision, and make an incision parallel to the direction of the hair to avoid cutting the hair roots.
6. Make an incision following Langer's lines.
7. Ensure the incision is of sufficient length for the surgery.

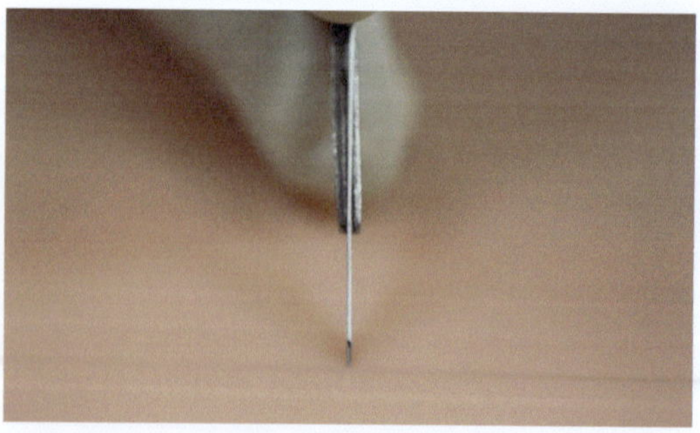

**Fig. 1.1** The blade starts at a right angle to the surface

8. Avoid anatomical structures such as nerves, blood vessels, etc.
9. Consider aesthetic aspects.
10. Consider the patient's unique condition (the existence of preexisting scars, injured areas).
11. When using a flap, avoid damaging the feeding vessels by suturing.

When placing an incision, careful consideration should be given to the location of nerves and vessels in the surgical site. For mucosal incisions, the same considerations as skin incisions are necessary in areas exposed to the outside such as the lip area. In other areas like the oral floor, palate, and submucosal tissues, it is essential to consider the direction of vessels, nerves, salivary ducts, and muscles to avoid damaging them. Accidental damage to these structures can lead to complications such as paresthesia, excessive bleeding, or even tissue necrosis. Therefore, a comprehensive understanding of the anatomy of the oral cavity, including bone, soft tissue, and vascular and neural structures, is indispensable.

Furthermore, it is crucial to consider the patient's specific conditions, such as the presence of any underlying disease or disorder that might affect the healing process or increase the likelihood of postoperative complications. For instance, when a patient has a preexisting scar in the oral cavity, it may be advantageous to utilize this area for the incision, thus minimizing additional tissue trauma. Similarly, in patients who have suffered oral trauma, incisions can be planned to use the damaged tissue as an access point to the wounded area, sparing the unaffected tissues.

### 1.2.2 Classification of Incisions

Broadly, incisions can be categorized into two types: envelope (or sulcular) and three-cornered (or triangular) incisions (Fig. 1.2).

1. Envelope incisions: This incision type is commonly used in simple extractions where there is minimal bone removal. It involves a horizontal cut along the sulcus of the tooth, thereby forming an "envelope" around the tooth.
2. Three-cornered incisions: Used in more complex cases, such as impacted teeth or when significant bone removal is anticipated, this incision provides greater access to the surgical site. It involves a sulcular incision and a vertical releasing incision, forming a triangular flap.

The choice between the two primarily hinges on the complexity of the extraction and the dentist's judgment.

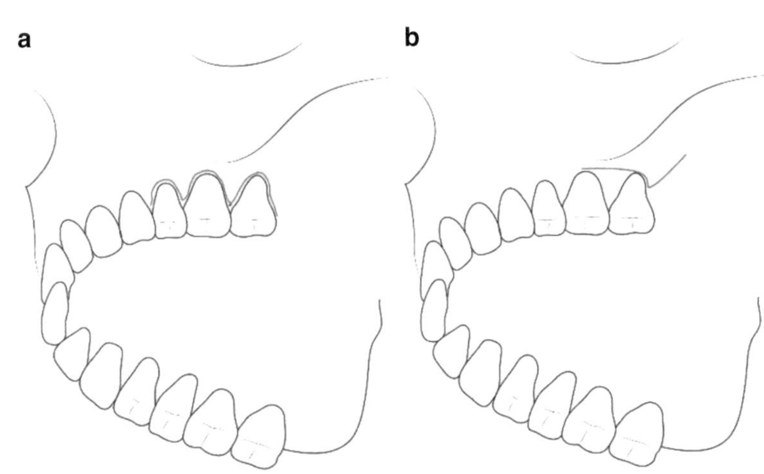


**Fig. 1.2** Design of incision. (**a**) envelope incision. (**b**) three-cornered incision

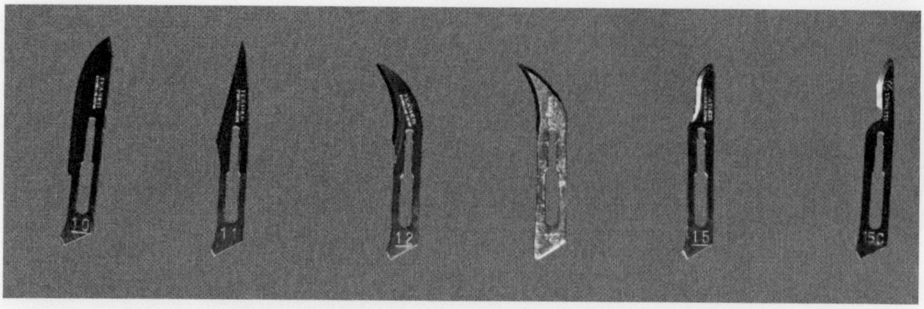

**Fig. 1.3** The scalpel blades. From left, No. 10, No. 11, No. 12, No. 12D, No. 15, and No. 15C

### 1.2.3 The Kind of Scalpel Blades

Regardless of the incision type, tooth extraction surgeries often result in what might be perceived as a "scalpel blade"—a disrupted oral environment characterized by the displacement of soft tissues, bone removal, and bleeding. Managing this "scalpel blade" is crucial in ensuring a smooth surgical procedure and optimal healing postoperation (Fig. 1.3).

In most intraoral surgeries, a #15 blade is commonly utilized. Its small, curved cutting edge allows for precise, delicate incisions, making it versatile for a variety of procedures, including tooth extraction. However, in situations where the area for incision is anatomically challenging, such as in the narrow interdental spaces or near the gingival margin, a #12 blade with its pointed, crescent-shaped edge may be more appropriate. This blade is specifically designed for making incisions in confined spaces and for periodontal and gingival surgeries. In contrast, when treating an abscess where a straight, puncture-style incision is required for drainage, a #11 blade is often the instrument of choice. Its long, straight, and pointed cutting edge makes it ideal for puncturing and draining abscesses.

Lastly, for longer incisions or when more extensive tissue removal is necessary, such as in some types of impacted tooth extraction, a #10 blade may be considered. Its larger, curved cutting edge is designed for making long, sweeping incisions.

In all cases, the proper scalpel holding technique is crucial (Fig. 1.4). There are two common grips: the "pen grip" and the "palm grip." The pen grip offers precision and control and is useful for delicate, shallow incisions. The palm grip, on the other hand, provides strength and stability, making it suitable for deeper, more forceful cuts. The choice of grip should be determined by the nature of the incision and the dentist's comfort level. Regardless of the grip, it is essential to always hold the scalpel with a steady hand, have a clear view of the surgical site, and make the incision with decisive, controlled movements. In all cases, safety should be the foremost concern—to avoid slips or accidental cuts, never use a scalpel in a way that feels unstable or uncomfortable.

This process involves various steps, starting with the gentle and careful retraction of the incised flap to minimize tissue damage. The removal of bone (if necessary) should be performed cautiously, and the extracted tooth needs to be handled with care to prevent any further damage. In all cases, it is essential to consider the nature of the procedure, the specific oral anatomy of the patient, and the surgeon's comfort with the blade in question when selecting the appropriate surgical instrument. The key takeaway is that while a certain degree of "scalpel blade" is an inherent part of surgical procedures, it can be effectively managed through appropriate planning, skilled execution, and careful postoperative care.

### 1.2.4 Bleeding Control

Bleeding control is an integral part of the incision process and overall surgical management. The source of bleeding should be swiftly identified and controlled using appropriate hemostatic tech-

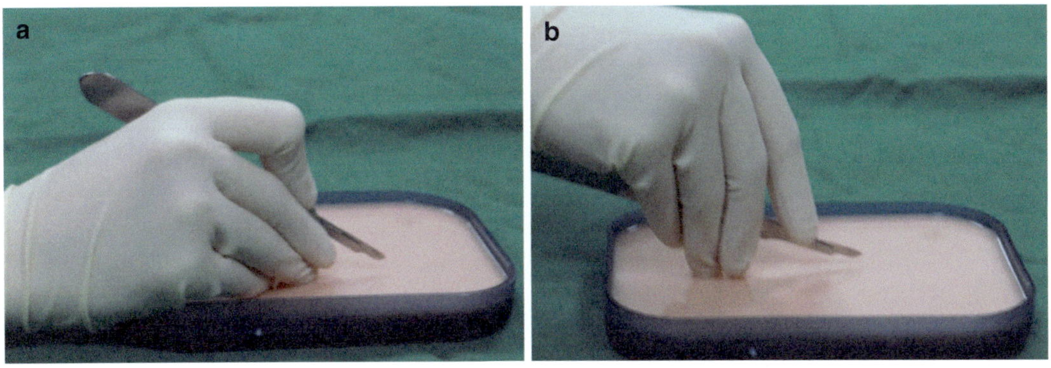


**Fig. 1.4** Scalpel holding technique. (**a**) pen grip and (**b**) palm grip

niques. These can include the use of pressure packs, hemostatic agents, sutures, or even electrocautery, depending on the severity and source of bleeding. The hemostatic agents can be enlisted as follows:

1. Epinephrine
2. Oxidized cellulose (Oxycel®, Surgicel®)
3. Microcrystalline collagen (Avitene®)
4. Absorbable gelatin sponge (Gelfoam®)
5. Tissue thromboplastin

The treatment of bleeding points during an incision can vary depending on whether the bleeding is capillary or due to the severing of small arteries or veins. For capillary bleeding, a mosquito-type hemostat can be used or a hemostatic agent can be applied. In the case of the severing of small arteries or veins, the blood vessels are clamped with a hemostat and then ligated or electrocauterized. Understanding that some amount of bleeding is normal and expected during and after tooth extraction can also help in setting appropriate patient expectations and in planning postoperative care. After tooth extraction, mild oozing from the extraction socket is common, even while biting down on gauze. This blood can mix with saliva, and if the patient spits it out, the clot in the extraction socket may be disrupted, leading to prolonged bleeding. Therefore, patients should swallow saliva while biting on gauze to aid in hemostasis.

In conclusion, the incision step, despite being the preliminary stage in tooth extraction, holds paramount importance. Mastery of incision techniques and principles is fundamental for dental practitioners to ensure the success of the extraction process and to minimize postoperative complications.

## 1.3 Suture

Suturing is an essential skill in oral surgery, used to close incisions and promote healing. It requires the understanding and correct application of several fundamental principles [2].

### 1.3.1 Classification of Needle

Needles used in dental surgery can be broadly classified into three categories: round-bodied, cutting, and reverse cutting (Fig. 1.5). Round-bodied needles are generally used for soft tissues as they separate rather than cut tissue. Cutting needles have a triangular cross-section and a sharp edge and are used for tougher tissue, like the oral mucosa. Reverse cutting needles are like cutting needles but have a cutting edge on the outer curve, reducing the risk of cutting through tissue.

### 1.3.2 The Requirement of Ideal Suture Material

Ideal suture materials should have several key properties: high tensile strength, good knot security, minimal tissue reaction, sterility, and if

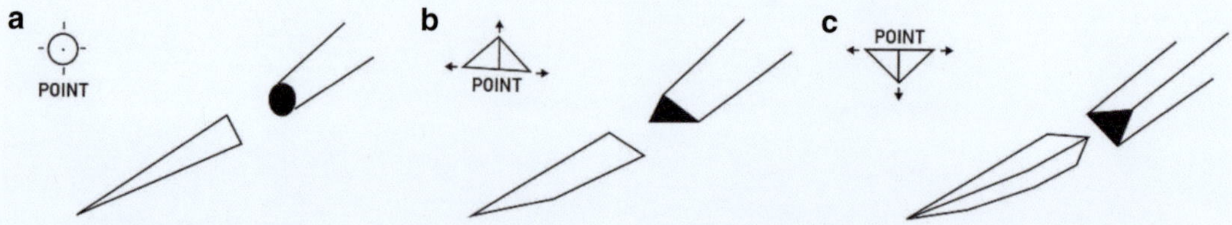


**Fig. 1.5** Classification of needle. (**a**) round-bodied, (**b**) cutting, and (**c**) reverse cutting

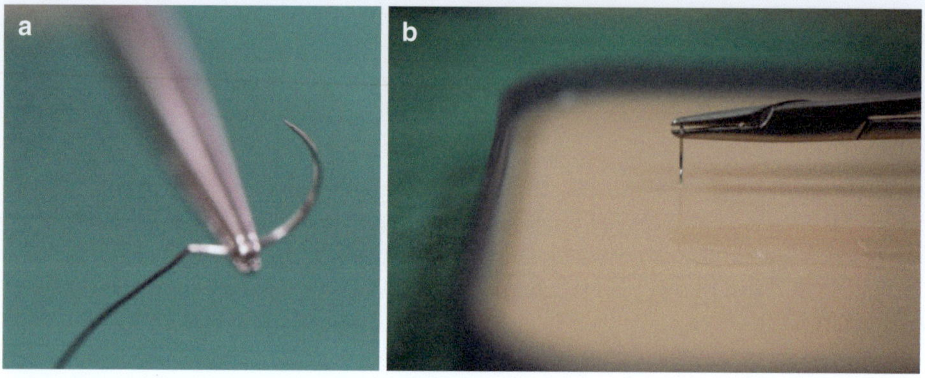


**Fig. 1.6** Managing a needle with a needle holder is a crucial technique in clinical settings. This process involves two primary steps: (**a**) grasping the suture needle using a needle holder and (**b**) ensuring that the suture needle enters the tissue perpendicular to the surface

required, slow absorbability. The selection of suture material is dependent on the type and location of the surgical procedure and the anticipated healing time.

1. It should have adequate tensile strength.
2. It should elicit minimal tissue reaction.
3. It should be nonelectrolytic.
4. It should not cause capillary action.
5. It should not cause hypersensitivity reactions.
6. It should be easy to handle (handle comfortably).
7. It should not be carcinogenic.
8. It should be able to be sterilized without undergoing physical changes.
9. It should be affordable.

### 1.3.3 The Principle of Suture

The guiding principle of suturing is to bring the wound edges together to promote healing, without causing undue pressure, inflammation, or damage. The suture should be placed at an equal distance from the wound edge at both the entry and exit points, with the knot resting against the tissue to prevent movement and potential tissue necrosis.

1. Grasp the suture needle at three-quarters from the tip with the needle holder (Fig. 1.6a).
2. The suture needle enters the tissue perpendicular to the surface (Fig. 1.6b).
3. The suture needle passes through the tissue according to its curvature.
4. The suture is located at the same distance from the incision and maintains the same depth.
5. In the case of a flap, suture from the free side to the fixed side.
6. If there is a difference in thickness between the two sides, the suture needle passes deeper through the thinner tissue.
7. The depth at which the needle enters the tissue should be greater than the distance from

the tissue edge, and the tissue should be slightly everted.
8. There should be no tension, and if necessary, undermine the tissue.
9. The tissues should be approximated only, not pulled too taut to cause blanching.
10. Do not place the knot on the incision line.
11. The spacing between sutures should be constant, around 3–4 mm.
12. Take measures to prevent the formation of a dog ear (a protrusion at the end of a suture line).

### 1.3.4 The Objective of Suture

The main objectives of suturing are to stop bleeding, stabilize the tissue to promote healing, minimize the risk of infection, reduce scar formation, and restore the function and aesthetics of the oral cavity.

### 1.3.5 The Size of Suture Material and Their Indications

Suture materials come in various sizes, typically ranging from 1-0 (or even larger sizes like 0, 00, etc.) to 10-0. The sizing can seem counterintuitive, as the larger the number before the dash (e.g., 10 in 10-0), the smaller the diameter of the suture material. This range in suture sizes allows for specific applications in various surgical scenarios, ensuring the appropriate strength and flexibility based on tissue type and location.

1. 1-0 to 3-0: These are thicker sutures and are commonly used in areas requiring greater tensile strength. Indications include:
   (a) Deep dermal sutures
   (b) Muscular layers
   (c) Palatal procedures in dental surgeries
2. 4-0 to 5-0: These are medium-sized sutures and find use in areas where a balance between strength and aesthetics is crucial. Indications include:
   (a) Superficial skin layers
   (b) Mucosal layers in oral surgeries
3. 6-0 to 7-0: These are fine sutures ideal for areas where minimal scarring is desirable. Indications include:
   (a) Delicate mucosal layers
   (b) Fine skin areas, such as the face
4. 8-0 to 10-0: These are ultrafine sutures used in microsurgical procedures. While less common in dental surgeries, their indications include:
   (a) Microvascular procedures
   (b) Ophthalmic surgeries

In dental surgeries, the choice of suture size will largely depend on the specific oral region being operated on, the type of tissue being sutured, and the expected tension on the sutured area. For instance, gingival or mucosal surgeries might prefer the use of 4-0 or 5-0 sizes, ensuring both strength and minimal scarring. Meanwhile, deeper oral procedures that involve muscle layers or palatal tissues might necessitate the use of 1-0 to 3-0 sizes for optimal tensile strength.

### 1.3.6 Classification of Suture Materials

Suture materials are broadly classified into two categories based on their ability to be broken down and absorbed by the body [3].

1. Absorbable sutures:
   (a) Description: These sutures are designed to degrade over time once they have been placed in the body. The degradation might result from enzymatic reactions or hydrolysis. As they degrade, their tensile strength decreases, eventually leaving no trace in the tissue.
   (b) Common materials: Catgut, polyglycolic acid, polylactic acid, polydioxanone, and others.
   (c) Indications:
      - Used primarily in internal suturing, especially where the presence of a suture material might interfere with function or might be bothersome if left indefinitely.

  - Beneficial in places that are hard to reach for suture removal.
  - Often chosen for oral surgeries, as they negate the need for a second procedure to remove sutures.

2. Nonabsorbable sutures:
   (a) Description: These sutures are made from materials that do not degrade within the tissue. They remain intact indefinitely unless removed. They maintain their tensile strength for a much longer duration.
   (b) Common materials: Nylon, polypropylene, silk, polyester, and stainless steel.
   (c) Indications:
   - Ideal for skin closures or any location where prolonged support is needed.
   - They are often removed once the tissue has healed sufficiently, although in some deep surgeries, they may be left in place.
   - In dental procedures, they can be used for procedures where the suture's prolonged presence will not adversely affect the outcome, or where its removal can be easily accomplished.

While both types of sutures have their distinct advantages, the choice between absorbable and nonabsorbable largely depends on the surgical context, the expected healing rate of the tissue, and the patient's comfort and needs. In dental surgeries, careful consideration of the procedure's nature and the postoperative care plan is crucial in making an appropriate choice.

### 1.3.7 The Method for Suture

There are several techniques for suturing, each with its uses (Fig. 1.7).

1. Single interrupted suture: This is the most used technique due to its versatility and reliability. Each stitch is made separately and tied off, allowing the removal of individual stitches without affecting the others.
2. Mattress suture: This technique is used to bring together large wound edges. It involves the placement of horizontal or vertical sutures that incorporate a larger area of tissue.
3. Three-point suture or four-point suture: This technique is used in areas where tension is high. It distributes the tension over three or four points, reducing the risk of tissue tearing.
4. Continuous suture: This is a quicker technique in which the suture is run continuously along the wound edge without being tied off after each pass. It is useful for long wounds but has the disadvantage that if the suture breaks, the entire line of suturing may come undone.
5. Locking continuous suture: This is like the continuous suture but has "locks" at each stitch, preventing the entire suture line from coming undone if the suture material breaks at any point.
6. Subcuticular suture: This technique is used for suturing the layer beneath the skin, minimizing scar visibility. The suture is placed in the dermis, so it is not visible on the skin surface.

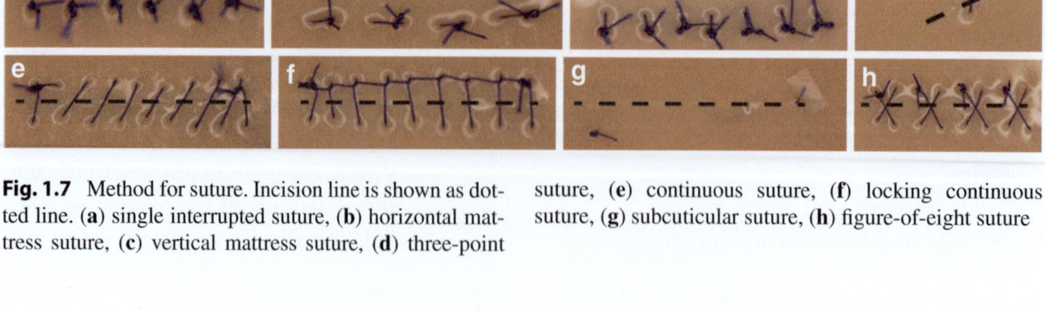


**Fig. 1.7** Method for suture. Incision line is shown as dotted line. (**a**) single interrupted suture, (**b**) horizontal mattress suture, (**c**) vertical mattress suture, (**d**) three-point suture, (**e**) continuous suture, (**f**) locking continuous suture, (**g**) subcuticular suture, (**h**) figure-of-eight suture

7. Figure-of-eight suture: This is used to close small, circular wounds or to tie off vessels. It involves the placement of sutures in a figure-of-eight pattern.

### 1.3.8 Knot

The knot secures the suture and ensures the wound edges stay together during healing. It should be tied securely, without causing ischemia or tissue necrosis. It should also be placed appropriately to minimize discomfort and prevent untimely dehiscence (Fig. 1.8).

1. Square knot (reef knot): This is the simplest and most used knot in surgical suturing. It is made by taking one end of a piece of string in each hand, crossing them, tucking one under the other, and pulling it tight (Fig. 1.8a). Then, the process is repeated in reverse, with the string that went under last time going over. The square knot is secure, and lies flat when properly tied, making it ideal for most suturing tasks. However, it is worth noting that it can become unstable under continuous pressure.
2. Granny knot: This knot is like a square knot, but less secure. It is created the same way as a square knot, except the crossover is not reversed for the second tie, meaning that the same end of the string goes under both times (Fig. 1.8b). This creates an unbalanced knot that tends to slip under pressure and is therefore not generally used in surgical applications.
3. Surgeon's knot: This is a modification of the square knot that adds an extra twist when tying the first throw, creating two overlapping loops (Fig. 1.8c). This provides additional friction that keeps the knot tight while the second throw is being tied, which can be particularly useful when dealing with slippery suture materials or when applying sutures in deep wounds. The second throw is then made as in the square knot, creating a secure, stable knot.

These are general descriptions of these knots. The exact technique for tying them can vary somewhat, and it is often worth learning from a demonstration or hands-on practice. In surgical practice, the choice of knot will often depend on the specific needs of the procedure and the preferences of the surgeon.

### 1.3.9 Timing for Stitch-Out

Stitches should be removed (stitch-out) as soon as possible, within the limits that do not allow the wound to dehisce. Wound dehiscence after suture removal indicates that the suture may have been removed too early. If spontaneous knot release and wound dehiscence occur, additional sutures should be placed as necessary.

1. 2–3 days: In areas where the dermis is thin and the blood supply is good.

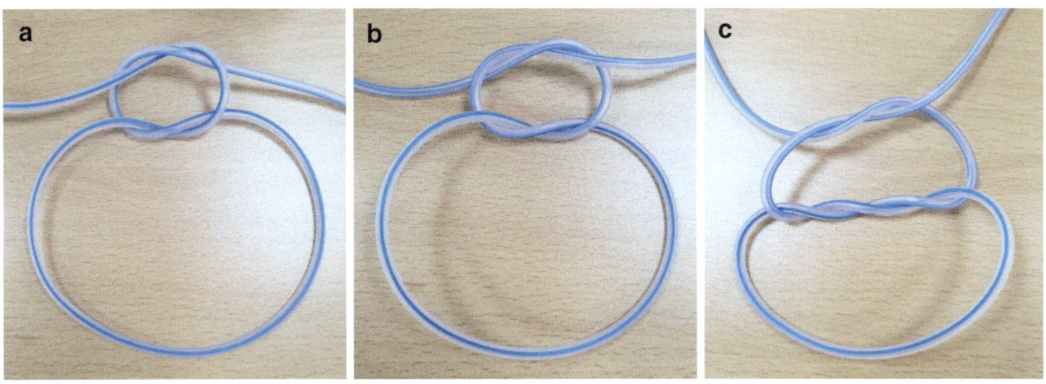


**Fig. 1.8** Knot. (**a**) square knot (reef knot), (**b**) granny knot, (**c**) surgeon's knot

2. 8–12 days: In areas where the dermis is thick and there is high tension.
3. Scalp 5–6 days, face 3–6 days, neck 5–7 days, trunk (anterior) 7–12 days, limbs 7–14 days.
4. Generally, stitches are kept for 7 days, and for the oral cavity, they are removed after 5–7 days.
5. To remove the suture, hold the suture with a tool, lift it above the epidermis, and then cut the side closer to the surface of the epidermis.
6. When removing the suture, prevent tension by pulling toward the wound.

It is crucial to remember that these are general guidelines and the exact timing for stitch removal can vary depending on several factors such as the individual's healing capacity, the location and size of the wound, and the suture material used. As always, professional judgment is needed for determining the appropriate stitch-out timing.

## 1.4 Dressing

1. The Aim of Dressing

   The primary aim of dressing after surgery is to protect the wound from external contaminants, to help in managing bleeding and exudate, to provide a conducive environment for the natural healing process, and to provide comfort and support to the patient [4].
2. The Requirement of Ideal Dressing

   The ideal dressing material should fulfill several criteria. It should be sterile to avoid introducing new sources of infection. The material should be absorbent enough to manage the exudate and any residual bleeding from the surgical site. It must be permeable to gases for proper tissue breathing but impermeable to bacteria to prevent infection. It should also provide a moist environment at the wound-dressing interface, promoting wound healing. Importantly, the dressing must be nonadherent to avoid causing trauma when being removed and should be easy to apply and remove.
3. Dressing for Closed Wound

   A closed wound often involves suturing and does not expose the underlying tissues and structures. For such wounds, a simple sterile dressing or surgical gauze is commonly used. The dressing is changed periodically, depending on the volume of exudate and the condition of the wound. During dressing changes, the wound should be inspected for signs of infection, such as increasing redness, swelling, pain, or discharge.
4. Dressing for Open Wound

   Open wounds, like those that might occur with complicated procedures or when a wound cannot be sutured, require specialized dressings. The dressing should ensure a moist wound environment conducive to healing and capable of absorbing a large volume of exudate. It should also conform to the wound surface for effective protection. A range of products, including alginate dressings, hydrocolloid dressings, and foam dressings, may be appropriate depending on the specific characteristics of the wound.

## 1.5 Conclusion

The intricate process of tooth extraction, especially in advanced scenarios, is more than just a simple removal. It requires a delicate combination of sound knowledge, dexterity, and an understanding of the surgical principles at play. From making the precise incision to understanding the significance of suturing techniques, every step holds paramount importance. Dressing, as the final step, not only protects the wound but also aids in healing, preventing potential complications.

Over the course of this chapter, we have explored the various aspects of surgical principles for advanced tooth extraction, understanding the depth and breadth of each stage. As we have seen, each stage has its own intricacies and challenges. Incorporating these principles into practice requires constant learning, patience, and experience. Each extraction is unique, and while these principles provide a foundation, adapting to the specific needs of each patient and situation is crucial.

## References


1. Sanz M, Simion M, Working Group 3 of the European Workshop on Periodontology. Surgical techniques on periodontal plastic surgery and soft tissue regeneration: consensus report of Group 3 of the 10th European Workshop on Periodontology. J Clin Periodontol. 2014;41 Suppl 15:S92–7. https://doi.org/10.1111/jcpe.12215.
2. Brandt MT, Jenkins WS. Suturing principles for the dentoalveolar surgeon. Dent Clin N Am. 2012;56(1):281–303. https://doi.org/10.1016/j.cden.2011.08.004.
3. Yag-Howard C. Sutures, needles, and tissue adhesives: a review for dermatologic surgery. Dermatologic Surg. 2014;40(Suppl 9):S3–S15. https://doi.org/10.1097/01.DSS.0000452738.23278.2d.
4. Trucillo P, Di Maio E. Classification and production of polymeric foams among the systems for wound treatment. Polymers. 2021;13(10):1608. https://doi.org/10.3390/polym13101608.

# Diagnostic Considerations for Complex Extraction Cases

2

## Contents



## 2.1 Introduction

Complex extraction cases in dentistry refer to scenarios where teeth require removal, but present significant challenges due to various anatomical, pathological, or patient-related factors. Unlike straightforward extractions, complex cases necessitate a higher level of expertise, meticulous planning, and often, interdisciplinary collaboration to ensure successful outcomes and minimize associated risks. Complex extraction cases are often delineated by the presence of one or more complicating factors that elevate the level of difficulty and risk involved in the extraction procedure. These factors may encompass abnormal tooth morphology, challenging tooth position, proximity to vital anatomical structures, or associated pathological conditions. The complexity might also be augmented by patient-related factors such as systemic diseases, medication use, or previous surgical history.

**Common Examples**

- Impacted teeth: Impaction refers to teeth that have failed to erupt into their correct position in the oral cavity due to lack of space, improper angulation, or other obstructions.
- Teeth associated with cysts or tumors: Teeth may be associated with cysts or tumors, which can complicate their extraction and may require additional surgical procedures.
- Teeth with extensive periapical pathology: Teeth with extensive periapical pathology


S.-G. Kim et al., *Advanced Strategies for Tooth Extraction in Dentistry*,
https://doi.org/10.1007/978-981-97-6532-4_2

often present challenges due to infection, bone loss, or other surrounding tissue damage.
- Anatomical challenges: Cases where teeth are near vital structures such as nerves, blood vessels, or the sinus cavity demand careful consideration and technique to avoid injury.

The prevalence of complex extraction cases can vary widely based on demographic factors, dental health awareness, and access to dental care among different populations. Common scenarios leading to complex extractions include neglected dental care, traumatic injuries, or congenital anomalies that result in abnormal tooth development or positioning. The potential risks and complications associated with complex extractions are multifaceted. They may include but are not limited to, postoperative infection, bleeding, damage to adjacent structures, prolonged healing, and the necessity for further surgical interventions. Additionally, complex extractions can also have a psychological impact on patients, who might experience anxiety or fear associated with the procedure.

Accurate diagnosis is foundational for the formulation of a comprehensive treatment plan in dental practice. It is especially crucial in complex extraction cases where a misdiagnosis can significantly impact the treatment outcome. An accurate diagnosis helps in understanding the exact nature and extent of the dental issue, which in turn aids in deciding the most appropriate treatment modality. Various treatment options such as vital pulp treatment, nonsurgical root canal treatment, surgical root canal treatment, extraction, or referral can be considered based on the accurate diagnosis of the dental condition [1].

A thorough patient assessment, encompassing a detailed medical and dental history, is paramount to arriving at an accurate diagnosis. This is often the first step in the diagnostic process and provides invaluable insights into the patient's overall health status and specific dental issues. A comprehensive patient history facilitates an accurate diagnosis, which is essential for devising an effective treatment plan. The treatment plan thus formulated is more likely to address the patient's dental issues adequately and ensure successful outcomes [2].

Diagnostic tools are indispensable in complex extraction cases. Among these, radiographic examination stands out as a vital tool, providing crucial information about the roots and surrounding tissues, thus aiding in the accurate assessment of the dental condition. While radiographic examination is widely acknowledged as important, its use before dental extraction is not universally implemented, suggesting a scope for standardization in diagnostic protocols [3]. Inaccurate or inadequate diagnosis can lead to improper treatment planning, which in turn can result in failed treatments, recurrent dental issues, and additional costs for the patient. For instance, without a complete understanding of the clinical situation, the true success of a restoration cannot be ensured, and the same issues are likely to arise again in the future. Accurate diagnosis and treatment planning following orthodontic extraction guidelines, for example, lead to long-term stability of the corrected results, emphasizing the significance of precision in the diagnostic phase [4].

The primary aim of this chapter is to equip readers with the requisite knowledge and understanding needed to effectively manage complex extraction cases. Through a thorough exploration of diagnostic considerations, readers will gain insights into the intricacies involved in handling such challenging dental scenarios. This chapter strives to provide a comprehensive overview of the factors that contribute to the complexity of certain extraction cases, the importance of accurate diagnosis, and the various imaging techniques that aid in treatment planning. By the end of this chapter, readers should have a solid foundation upon which to build their diagnostic acumen and clinical skills in managing complex extraction cases.

Understanding the diagnostic considerations in managing complex extraction cases is pivotal for ensuring successful outcomes and minimizing potential complications. The knowledge imparted in this chapter aims to enhance the reader's ability to accurately diagnose and plan treatments for complex extraction scenarios. Emphasis is placed on the significance of a thorough preoperative assessment, the utilization of appropriate imaging techniques, and the formulation of a well-thoughtout treatment plan based on accurate diagnosis.

This subsection serves as a segue into the more detailed discussions in the following sections of the chapter. It sets the stage for a deeper dive into the general factors associated with extraction, past medical history considerations, imaging techniques, and other pertinent topics. The subsequent sections aim to further elucidate the diagnostic and management considerations essential for dealing with complex extraction cases, thereby providing a more granular understanding of the subject matter. The objective is to foster a well-rounded comprehension of the multifaceted nature of complex extraction cases, thereby better preparing the reader to handle such cases in clinical practice.

## 2.2 Preoperative Assessment

The preoperative assessment is a critical component in managing complex extraction cases. This assessment lays the groundwork for a safe and effective treatment plan. It typically includes a clinical examination, a thorough review of the patient's medical and dental history, and a detailed patient consultation, culminating in informed consent. Each of these components plays a vital role in the overall process.

1. Clinical Examination

   The clinical examination is the first step in the preoperative assessment. It involves a comprehensive evaluation of the patient's oral cavity and related structures. This examination should focus on

   - Oral inspection: Examine the oral mucosa, gingival tissues, and the condition of the teeth, including their alignment, presence of decay, and any signs of infection.
   - Periodontal assessment: Evaluate the health of the gums and supporting bone structure. Note any signs of periodontal disease which may affect the extraction procedure.
   - Occlusal evaluation: Assess the patient's bite and look for any occlusal anomalies that might impact the extraction and subsequent healing.
   - Palpation: Feel the soft tissues, including the lymph nodes and salivary glands, to check for abnormalities.

2. Review of Medical and Dental History

   This part of the assessment is crucial for identifying any underlying health conditions that might affect the extraction process:

   - Medical history: Gather information about the patient's general health, including past surgeries, chronic illnesses (like diabetes or hypertension), allergies, and current medications. This information helps in identifying potential complications and planning for them.
   - Dental history: Review the patient's dental history, focusing on previous dental treatments and surgeries. This helps in understanding the patient's dental health trajectory and any recurrent issues.

3. Patient Consultation and Informed Consent

   The final step in the preoperative assessment is a thorough patient consultation, followed by obtaining informed consent:

   - Consultation: Engage in a detailed discussion with the patient. This includes understanding their expectations, addressing their concerns, and explaining the risks and benefits of the procedure. This conversation helps in building a rapport and trust with the patient.
   - Risk identification: Discuss any potential risk factors identified during the clinical examination and history review. This might include risks associated with the patient's specific health conditions, medication interactions, or complexities identified in the oral examination.
   - Informed consent: Ensure that the patient understands all aspects of the procedure, including potential complications and

postoperative care. Informed consent should be obtained in writing, confirming that the patient comprehends the procedure and consents to it willingly.

Throughout the preoperative assessment, the dentist must maintain an empathetic and professional approach, ensuring that the patient feels heard and understood. This comprehensive assessment not only aids in the safe execution of the extraction but also helps in building a trusting relationship with the patient, which is vital for successful treatment outcomes.

## 2.3 General Factors Associated with Extraction

This section explores the various general factors that significantly influence the complexity and approach to tooth extractions. Understanding these factors is key to effective treatment planning and successful outcomes. The subsections focus on anatomical considerations, the condition of the tooth and surrounding tissues, and the influence of patient age and systemic health.

1. Anatomical Considerations
   - Complex root structures: Teeth with curved, multi-rooted, or unusually long roots pose challenges in extraction. Careful evaluation using imaging techniques is essential to map out these structures.
   - Proximity to critical anatomy: The proximity of teeth to nerves, sinuses, and blood vessels can increase the risk of complications. For the extraction of maxillary molars and premolars, assessing maxillary sinus pneumatization is crucial to prevent accidental displacement of the tooth into the sinus. For mandibular third molar surgery, confirming the location of the inferior alveolar nerve and lingual nerve is essential to avoid nerve damage. When a mandibular third molar is ankylosed to the lingual plate, its extraction may lead to a fracture of the lingual plate, which could, in turn, risk damage to the lingual artery. Precise imaging and surgical planning are necessary to minimize risks.
   - Bone density and access: Dense bone or limited access in the oral cavity, such as in the case of impaction, complicates extractions. These factors require specific surgical techniques and equipment.

   Guidelines
   - Utilize detailed imaging to assess anatomical challenges.
   - Plan for potential complications based on the anatomical analysis.
   - Consider referral to specialists in cases of high-risk anatomical proximity.
2. Tooth Condition and Surrounding Tissue Health
   - Periodontal disease: Advanced periodontal disease can lead to weakened support for teeth, complicating extractions. When a patient wishes to extract some, but not all, teeth affected by periodontal disease, the remaining teeth may eventually exfoliate on their own. To prevent any legal complications, this possibility should be clearly communicated to the patient.
   - Tooth decay and fracture: Severely decayed or fractured teeth may not be amenable to standard extraction techniques and may require surgical intervention. In cases of mesially inclined mandibular third molars, proximal caries frequently develops on the distal surface of the mandibular second molar. During extraction, there is a risk of partial crown fracture of the second molar. This possibility should be communicated to the patient prior to third molar extraction.
   - Infection and inflammation: Active infection or inflammation can increase the complexity of the procedure and the risk of postoperative complications.

   Guidelines
   - Assess the extent of decay or damage and plan the extraction method accordingly.
   - Prepare for potential surgical interventions in cases of severe tooth condition.
   - Address active infections or inflammation before proceeding with extraction.

3. Patient Age and Systemic Health
   - Elderly patients: Age-related factors like bone density loss and medical comorbidities can impact the extraction process and healing. Research cited in American Association of Oral and Maxillofacial Surgeons (AAOMS) guidelines suggests that patients over the age of 25–26 may have a higher risk of complications, including increased difficulty of extraction, prolonged healing times, and greater susceptibility to nerve injury or postoperative infections.
   - Pediatric patients: In younger patients, considerations include the stage of dental development and the impact on future dental alignment.
   - Systemic health conditions: Conditions such as diabetes, osteoporosis, or autoimmune diseases can affect healing and response to treatment.

Guidelines
   - Tailor extraction techniques to suit age-related dental and bone conditions.
   - Consult with the patient's healthcare providers to understand the implications of systemic health conditions.
   - Adjust postoperative care plans to accommodate age and health-related healing capacities.

In conclusion, these general factors play a pivotal role in the complexity of tooth extractions. A thorough understanding and strategic approach to these factors are essential for minimizing risks and ensuring effective treatment outcomes. Dentists should integrate these considerations into their treatment planning, adapting their techniques and strategies to the unique challenges presented by each case.

## 2.4 Past Medical History Associated with Extraction

The review of a patient's past medical history is a crucial step in preparing for a dental extraction, especially in complex cases. This review helps in identifying potential risk factors that could complicate the extraction process or impact postoperative recovery. The history should encompass systemic diseases, medication history, and previous surgical experiences, each of which can have significant implications for dental procedures.

1. Systemic Diseases Affecting Extraction
   - Diabetes: Patients with diabetes, especially those with poor glycemic control, may have an increased risk of infection and delayed healing. Monitoring blood sugar levels and coordinating care with the patient's primary physician may be necessary.
   - Hypertension: High blood pressure can increase the risk of bleeding during and after the extraction. It is important to ensure that hypertension is well-controlled prior to the procedure.
   - Bleeding disorders: Conditions like hemophilia or chronic anticoagulant therapy can lead to excessive bleeding. Preoperative planning may involve adjusting medication regimens or coordinating care with a hematologist.
   - Other systemic conditions: Conditions such as osteoporosis, autoimmune diseases, and chronic respiratory diseases also need to be considered as they can affect treatment planning and postoperative care.
2. Medication History and Potential Interactions
   - Anticoagulants and antiplatelet agents: These medications increase the risk of bleeding. Collaboration with the patient's healthcare provider is essential to manage these risks while minimizing the potential for thrombotic complications.
   - Bisphosphonates: Commonly used in osteoporosis, these drugs can affect bone healing and increase the risk of osteonecrosis, particularly after invasive procedures like tooth extractions.
   - Immunosuppressants: Patients on immunosuppressant therapy may have a heightened risk of infection, necessitating a more cautious approach and possibly prophylactic antibiotics.

3. Previous Surgeries and Anesthesia Considerations
   - Anesthetic reactions: A history of adverse reactions to anesthesia requires careful selection of anesthetic agents and techniques.
   - Surgical history: Previous surgeries, especially those involving the head, neck, or oral cavity, can impact the current extraction procedure due to changes in anatomy or scar tissue.
   - Anesthesia in systemic diseases: Patients with systemic diseases may require special consideration in anesthesia choice to avoid exacerbating their condition. For example, patients with respiratory diseases might require careful monitoring to prevent respiratory depression under sedation.
4. Integrating Medical History into Dental Care
   - Interdisciplinary communication: Effective communication with the patient's other healthcare providers is often necessary for a comprehensive understanding of the patient's health status and safe management of their dental needs.
   - Customizing anesthesia and pain management: The choice of anesthesia and postoperative pain management should be tailored to the patient's medical history, considering any potential interactions with existing medications and health conditions.
   - Postoperative monitoring: Patients with certain systemic conditions or those on specific medications may require more intensive postoperative monitoring and follow-up to mitigate risks such as infection, poor wound healing, or bleeding.

In summary, a detailed review of the patient's past medical history is indispensable for safely conducting dental extractions, particularly in complex cases. This review helps in identifying and mitigating potential risks associated with systemic diseases, medication interactions, and previous surgical experiences, thereby ensuring a safer and more effective extraction process.

## 2.5 Imaging Techniques

The use of imaging techniques in dental practice, especially for complex extractions, is indispensable. These techniques provide critical information about the tooth, its position, root morphology, and its relationship with surrounding anatomical structures. This section covers the types of imaging techniques used, how to interpret imaging findings, and the importance of imaging in treatment planning.

1. Types of Imaging Techniques
   - X-rays: The most common form of dental imaging, X-rays provide essential information about tooth decay, bone loss, and some aspects of root structure. They are quick, cost-effective, and widely available (Fig. 2.1).
   - Computed tomography (CT) scans: CT scans offer a more detailed view, presenting a three-dimensional image of the teeth, bones, and soft tissues. They are particularly useful for assessing complex cases such as impacted teeth, bone pathology, and precise location relative to nerves and sinuses.
   - Magnetic resonance imaging (MRI): While not commonly used for routine dental extractions, MRI can be invaluable in specific cases, particularly when soft tissue evaluation is necessary, such as in the case of cysts or tumors.
2. Recent Advancements
   - Digital and 3D imaging: Advances in digital technology have led to more precise imaging, often with lower radiation doses. 3D imaging techniques, such as cone-beam computed tomography (CBCT), provide detailed views of dental structures, aiding in more accurate treatment planning (Fig. 2.2).
3. Interpretation of Imaging Findings
   - Analyzing root morphology: Imaging helps in understanding the number, length, and curvature of roots, which is vital for planning extractions.

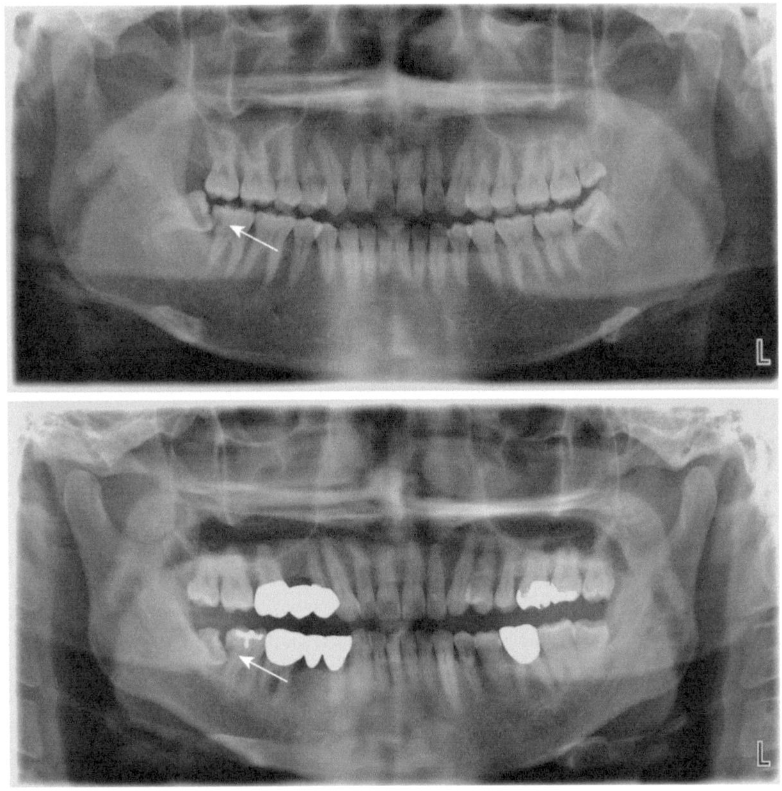

**Fig. 2.1** Panoramic radiogram. Dental caries is found in the second molar (arrows)

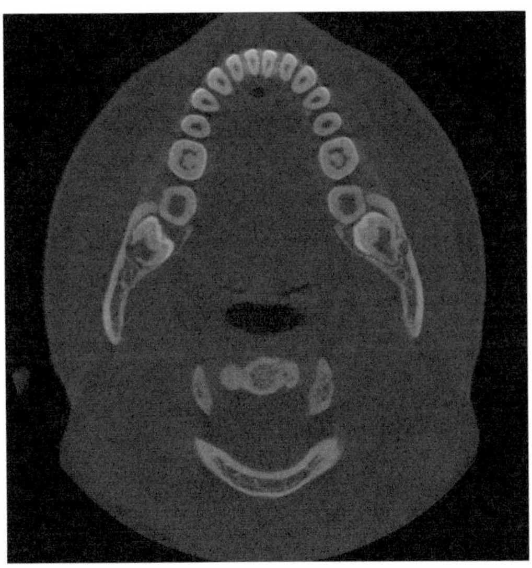

**Fig. 2.2** Cone-beam computed tomography (CBCT) image is used for the localization of the inferior alveolar nerve

- Identifying anatomical relationships: Imaging is crucial in determining the proximity of teeth to vital structures like nerves and sinuses, reducing the risk of inadvertent damage during extraction.
- Detecting pathologies: Imaging can reveal hidden dental pathologies like periapical infections, cysts, or tumors, which might alter the course of treatment.

4. Importance of Imaging in Treatment
   - Customizing surgical approaches: With detailed imaging, dental surgeons can customize their surgical approach to minimize trauma and optimize outcomes.
   - Preoperative planning: Imaging helps in creating a comprehensive preoperative plan, reducing the likelihood of unexpected complications during extraction.

- Patient education and consent: Imaging findings can be used to educate patients about their condition and the proposed treatment plan, facilitating informed consent.

Imaging techniques are a cornerstone in the diagnosis and treatment planning of complex dental extractions. The choice of imaging technique depends on the specific requirements of each case. Advances in imaging technology continue to enhance the precision and safety of dental extractions, contributing significantly to successful patient outcomes. Understanding and effectively interpreting these imaging findings is crucial for dental professionals in the planning and execution of complex extraction procedures.

## 2.6 Special Considerations

In the realm of complex dental extractions, certain patient populations and specific dental conditions require special consideration. This section addresses the management of anxious patients, the care of patients with special needs, and the treatment of medically compromised individuals. These considerations are vital for ensuring patient comfort and safety, as well as for the success of the extraction procedure.

1. Management of Anxious Patients
   - Understanding patient anxiety: Dental anxiety or phobia is common and can significantly impact patient cooperation and the success of the procedure. Understanding the root of this anxiety is the first step in effective management.
   - Communication strategies: Clear, empathetic communication about the procedure can alleviate fears. Providing detailed explanations and addressing concerns can help in building trust.
   - Sedation options: For highly anxious patients, various sedation methods, from mild anxiolytics to IV sedation or general anesthesia, can be considered depending on the severity of anxiety and the complexity of the procedure.
2. Patients with Special Needs
   - Pediatric patients: Children may require special attention to manage anxiety and ensure cooperation. Techniques like "tell-show-do" and the use of sedation or general anesthesia can be beneficial.
   - Geriatric patients: Older patients might have multiple comorbidities or cognitive impairments that require adjustments in treatment planning and patient management.
   - Physical and cognitive disabilities: Patients with disabilities may require modifications in approach, additional support, or specialized equipment. Coordination with caregivers and other healthcare providers is often necessary for effective treatment.
3. Medically Compromised Patients
   - Impacted teeth and complex cases: For teeth that are impacted or associated with cysts, tumors, or vital structures, a more cautious and meticulous surgical approach is necessary. Preoperative imaging and planning are crucial.
   - Patients with systemic diseases: Conditions like diabetes, heart disease, or bleeding disorders necessitate a tailored approach, often involving preoperative optimization of their medical condition and close postoperative monitoring.
   - Pain control: Effective pain management is crucial, particularly for medically compromised patients. The choice of analgesics should consider the patient's overall health status and any concurrent medications.

In summary, special considerations in complex dental extractions involve understanding and addressing the unique needs of various patient populations, including those with dental anxiety, special needs, and medical comorbidities. Additionally, the management of complex dental conditions such as impacted teeth or those associated with pathologies requires careful planning and execution. By adopting patient-centered approaches and utilizing appropriate management strategies, dental professionals can ensure safe, effective, and compassionate care for all patients undergoing complex dental extractions.

## 2.7 Treatment Planning

Effective treatment planning is a cornerstone in the management of complex dental extraction cases. This meticulous process involves formulating a comprehensive plan, thoroughly discussing risks and alternatives with the patient, and coordinating with other dental and medical professionals. This tailored approach ensures that each patient receives the most appropriate and effective care based on their unique clinical situation.

1. Formulating a Comprehensive Treatment Plan
   - Individualized approach: Every patient's situation is unique, and treatment plans should be customized based on their specific needs. This involves integrating findings from the clinical examination, imaging studies, and medical history.
   - Selection of extraction techniques: The choice of extraction technique, whether simple, surgical, or more specialized methods like piezoelectric extraction, depends on various factors such as tooth anatomy, the extent of impaction, and the proximity of vital structures. The treatment plan should outline the chosen technique and the rationale behind it.
   - Consideration of adjunctive procedures: In some cases, adjunct procedures like bone grafting or soft tissue management may be necessary. These should be included in the treatment plan when indicated.
2. Discussing Risks, Benefits, and Alternatives with the Patient
   - Informed consent: A key part of treatment planning is ensuring that the patient is fully informed about the risks, benefits, and potential alternatives to the proposed extraction. This discussion should be conducted in a manner that the patient can understand, accommodating any language or cognitive barriers.
   - Setting realistic expectations: It is important to set realistic expectations regarding the outcomes, potential complications, and the recovery process. This includes discussing the likelihood of success and the potential need for follow-up treatments.
   - Documentation: The discussions and the patient's decisions should be thoroughly documented in their medical record for legal and clinical purposes.
3. Coordination with Other Dental and Medical Professionals
   - Interdisciplinary collaboration: Complex extraction cases often require collaboration between various specialists such as oral surgeons, periodontists, prosthodontists, and even medical professionals like cardiologists or endocrinologists.
   - Referral considerations: In cases where the dentist feels a referral to a specialist is necessary, this should be discussed with the patient and coordinated efficiently.
   - Post-extraction follow-up: Coordination of post-extraction care, including follow-up appointments and management of any complications, is vital. This may involve both dental and medical professionals, depending on the patient's condition.

Treatment planning for complex dental extractions demands a comprehensive, patient-centered approach. This process involves careful consideration of the patient's unique clinical situation, clear communication about the proposed treatment, and close collaboration with other professionals. By adhering to these principles, dental practitioners can ensure that they provide the highest standard of care, tailored to the individual needs of each patient, thereby optimizing treatment outcomes and patient satisfaction.

## 2.8 Conclusion

The intricate process of tooth extraction, especially in advanced scenarios, is more than just a simple removal. It requires a delicate combination of sound knowledge, dexterity, and an understanding of the surgical principles at play. From making the precise incision to understanding the significance of suturing techniques, every step holds paramount importance. Dressing, as the final step, not only protects the wound but also aids in healing, preventing potential complications.

Over the course of this chapter, we have explored the various aspects of surgical principles for advanced tooth extraction, understanding the depth and breadth of each stage. As we have seen, each stage has its own intricacies and challenges. Incorporating these principles into practice requires constant learning, patience, and experience. Each extraction is unique, and while these principles provide a foundation, adapting to the specific needs of each patient and situation is crucial.

## References

1. Newsome P, Smales R, Yip K. Oral diagnosis and treatment planning: part 1. Introduction. Br Dent J. 2012;213(1):15–9. https://doi.org/10.1038/sj.bdj.2012.559.
2. Erian D, Quek SYP, Subramanian G. The importance of the history and clinical examination. J Am Dent Assoc. 2018;149(9):807–14. https://doi.org/10.1016/j.adaj.2017.12.019.
3. Talib Jiboon A, Alhamdani FY, Hussein Ali N. Radiographic examination before dental extraction from dentists' perspective. Int J Dent. 2023;2023:4970981. https://doi.org/10.1155/2023/4970981.
4. Al-Ani MH, Mageet AO. Extraction planning in orthodontics. J Contemp Dent Pract. 2018;19(5):619–23.

# 3 Techniques for Simple Extraction

## Contents



## 3.1 Introduction

Tooth extraction, a common dental procedure, involves the removal of a tooth from its socket in the bone. While it might seem straightforward, tooth extraction is a significant procedure in dental practice due to its implications for patient health and oral hygiene. The reasons for extracting a tooth vary, ranging from severe tooth decay, gum disease, to impacted wisdom teeth, and preparation for orthodontic treatment. The primary goal of tooth extraction is to alleviate pain, prevent the spread of infection, and maintain or improve oral health. It is a procedure that requires careful consideration, precise execution, and understanding of dental anatomy and patient health.

Tooth extractions are generally categorized into two types: simple and surgical. Simple extractions are performed on teeth that are visible in the mouth, typically under local anesthesia. These extractions are straightforward; the tooth is loosened and then removed with dental forceps. The process is relatively quick and usually has minimal complications. In contrast, surgical extractions involve removing teeth that are not easily accessible or visible. This could be because they have broken under the gum line or have not erupted fully, such as impacted wisdom teeth. Surgical extractions require more complex procedures, often involving incisions in the gum to access and remove the tooth or teeth. They may necessitate stronger anesthesia or sedation and generally have a longer recovery period.


S.-G. Kim et al., *Advanced Strategies for Tooth Extraction in Dentistry*,
https://doi.org/10.1007/978-981-97-6532-4_3

Mastering simple extraction techniques is crucial for dental practitioners. These techniques form the foundation for more complex dental surgeries and are frequently utilized in everyday dental practice. Effective simple extraction methods ensure minimal trauma to surrounding tissues, reduce patient discomfort, and speed up recovery times. Furthermore, understanding the nuances of simple extractions, such as identifying the right technique for different tooth types and positions, is essential for preventing complications. This knowledge also aids in educating patients about the procedure, managing their expectations, and providing effective aftercare instructions. Thus, simple tooth extraction, while routine, is a critical skill in dentistry, contributing significantly to patient care and oral health management.

## 3.2 Indications for Simple Tooth Extraction

1. Criteria for Selecting Simple Extraction: Tooth Condition and Patient Factors

   Simple tooth extractions are typically indicated when a tooth is irreparably damaged due to decay or trauma but remains visible and accessible in the mouth. The criteria for selecting a tooth for simple extraction involves assessing both the condition of the tooth and specific patient factors.

   (a) Tooth condition: The primary consideration is the state of the tooth. Teeth that are suitable for simple extraction generally have enough structural integrity to be removed in one piece. These teeth should not be fractured below the gum line, excessively mobile, or deeply impacted within the bone. The root structure of the tooth also plays a significant role. Teeth with a single, straight root, such as incisors, are often easier to extract than molars, which may have multiple roots with complex configurations. Conditions such as advanced periodontal disease, which can loosen the tooth's attachment to the surrounding bone, may facilitate a simple extraction.

   (b) Patient factors: The overall health and specific medical history of the patient are equally important. Systemic health conditions like diabetes or heart disease may impact the decision to proceed with an extraction, as well as the choice of anesthesia. Dentists must also consider factors like the patient's age, as the bone density in older patients may affect the ease of extraction. The patient's medication history, especially the use of bisphosphonates or anticoagulants, can influence the extraction process and postoperative healing.

2. Common Scenarios Requiring Simple Extraction

   There are several scenarios in which simple extraction is commonly required [1, 2]:

   (a) Decay: Severe decay that has destroyed significant portions of the tooth structure may necessitate extraction, especially if the decay has reached the pulp or caused infection.

   (b) Overcrowding: Orthodontic treatment often requires the removal of one or more teeth to create space for alignment, particularly in cases of dental overcrowding.

   (c) Periodontal disease: Advanced gum disease can lead to the loosening of teeth, making simple extraction necessary to prevent further oral health complications.

   (d) Non-restorable teeth: Teeth that cannot be restored due to extensive damage or poor prognosis, such as those with large fractures, can be candidates for simple extraction.

   (e) Primary teeth retention: In some cases, primary (baby) teeth do not fall out in time to allow the proper eruption of permanent teeth, requiring extraction.

   (f) Wisdom teeth: Early-stage problems with wisdom teeth, such as partial eruption or minor impaction, might be addressed with simple extraction in some cases.

## 3.3 Pre-Extraction Assessment

1. Patient Medical History Evaluation

   Before proceeding with a tooth extraction, a thorough evaluation of the patient's medical history is crucial. This assessment helps in identifying any underlying health conditions or medications that could affect the extraction procedure and post-extraction healing.

   (a) General health conditions: Conditions such as diabetes, heart disease, hypertension, and immune disorders can impact the patient's response to the extraction and healing. For example, diabetic patients may have delayed healing, and those with heart conditions may require antibiotic prophylaxis to prevent endocarditis [3].

   (b) Medications: It is vital to know the medications the patient is taking, particularly blood thinners like warfarin or aspirin, which can increase the risk of bleeding [4]. Patients on antiresorptive drugs like bisphosphonates and denosumab or anti-angiogenic drugs, for osteoporosis and cancer are at risk for osteonecrosis of the jaw, a serious condition that needs special consideration [5].

   (c) Allergies: Knowledge of any allergies, especially to local anesthetics or antibiotics, is essential to prevent adverse reactions during or after the procedure.

   (d) Previous dental history: Information about previous dental procedures and their outcomes can provide insights into how the patient might respond to the extraction.

2. Dental Examination: X-rays and Physical Inspection

   A comprehensive dental examination is the next step in pre-extraction assessment.

   (a) X-rays: Dental X-rays are indispensable for assessing the position, length, and condition of the root of the tooth to be extracted, as well as the proximity to neighboring teeth and anatomical structures like nerves and sinuses. They help in planning the extraction method and anticipating potential complications.

   (b) Physical inspection: A visual and tactile examination of the tooth and surrounding tissues is performed to assess the extent of decay, infection, and gum health. The dentist also checks for signs of periodontal disease, which may affect the extraction procedure.

3. Preparing the Patient: Addressing Anxiety and Pain Management

   Patient preparation is not only about the physical aspects but also involves addressing the psychological state of the patient.

   (a) Managing anxiety: Dental anxiety is common, and managing it is crucial for a smooth procedure. This can involve explaining the procedure in detail to the patient, using calming techniques, or, in some cases, sedation.

   (b) Pain management: Discussing pain management strategies beforehand is important. Local anesthesia is typically used to numb the area around the tooth to be extracted. The dentist might also discuss post-extraction pain relief options, including over-the-counter painkillers and prescription medications.

   (c) Post-extraction instructions: Providing clear instructions on what to expect after the extraction and how to care for the extraction site helps in preparing the patient mentally and can lead to better compliance and faster recovery.

## 3.4 Instrumentation and Materials

1. Overview of Tools Used in Simple Extractions (Elevators, Forceps)

   Simple tooth extractions primarily utilize two types of instruments: elevators and forceps. Understanding the function and design of these tools is essential for effective and safe extractions.

(a) Elevators

Elevators are instruments used to luxate, or loosen, the tooth from the periodontal ligament and ease its removal. They come in various shapes and sizes, each designed for specific applications. Common types include straight elevators, which are used to apply leverage against the tooth, and curved elevators, crafted with a curved design and paired in sets of two (for the left and right). Specialized elevators, like root tip picks, are designed to remove fractured root tips.

- Straight elevators (Fig. 3.1): These are the most common type of elevators. They are used to apply leverage against the tooth to loosen it from the periodontal ligament. Straight elevators are particularly effective for teeth with straight roots or when there is sufficient space to apply leverage.
- Curved elevators (Fig. 3.2): These elevators come in left and right variants and are used for elevating and loosening teeth. They are designed with a curved shape, allowing for better access to teeth at different angles.
- Root tip picks (Fig. 3.3): These are specialized elevators designed to remove root tips or fragments that may remain in the socket after the extraction of a broken tooth with left, right, and straight variants. Their fine tips and delicate structure allow for precise manipulation in tight spaces.
- Cryer elevators: Named after their inventor, these are used to remove roots or teeth in difficult positions, such as molars in the lower jaw. They are designed with a curved tip that fits around the tooth, providing leverage to lift the tooth out of its socket.
- Luxators: These are thin, sharp elevators used to cut the periodontal ligament and expand the bony socket. They are particularly useful for extracting teeth with minimal damage to surrounding tissues.

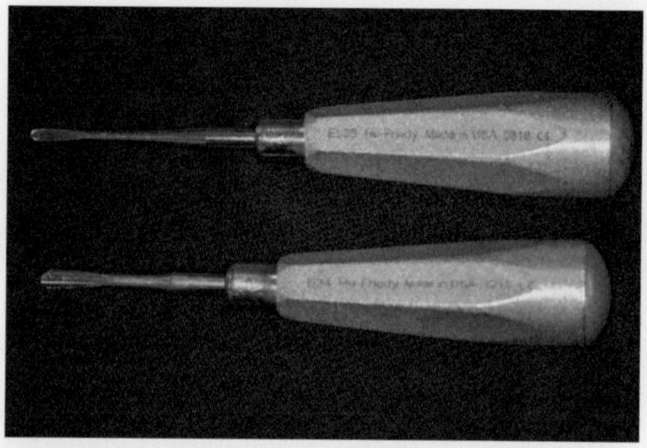

**Fig. 3.1** Straight elevator. The size of the blade varies

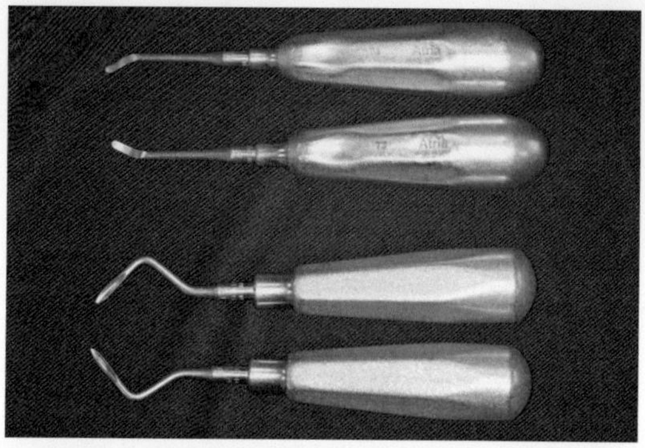

**Fig. 3.2** Curved elevator. There are left and right variants

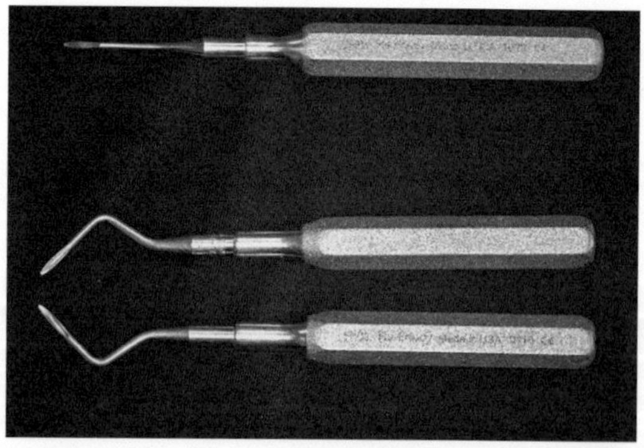

**Fig. 3.3** Root tip picks. There are left, right, and straight variants

(b) Forceps

Dental forceps are used to grasp and extract the tooth. Like elevators, they come in numerous designs, each tailored to specific teeth. For example, maxillary forceps typically have a beak that is angled to conform to the curve of the upper jaw, while mandibular forceps have a straighter design for the lower jaw. The beaks of the forceps are also designed according to the shape of the tooth; for instance, forceps for molars have broader and more curved beaks to accommodate the larger, multi-rooted tooth structure.

- Maxillary forceps: These are used for extracting teeth in the upper jaw. They come in various designs, each suited to different teeth:
  - Universal maxillary forceps (No. 150) (Fig. 3.4): Suitable for extracting premolars and molars, except for the third molars.
  - Maxillary anterior forceps (No. 1 or No. 99) (Fig. 3.5): Designed for incisors and canines, with a more delicate beak to grip these smaller teeth.
  - Maxillary molar forceps (No. 53, No. 88, or No. 210S) (Fig. 3.6): Specifically designed for upper molars, often with a right-angle design to accommodate the larger, multi-rooted structure of these teeth.
- Mandibular forceps: These are used for the lower jaw and have designs specific to this region:
  - Universal mandibular forceps (No. 151) (Fig. 3.7): Versatile for extracting premolars and molars, but not suitable for lower third molars.
  - Mandibular anterior forceps (No. 74 or No. 151A) (Fig. 3.8): Tailored for incisors and canines in the lower jaw, with a design that allows for a firm grip on these teeth.

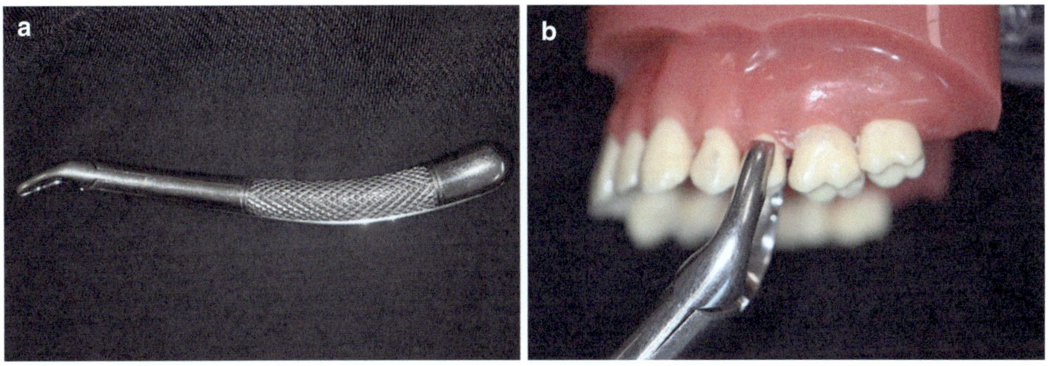


**Fig. 3.4** (**a**) Universal maxillary forceps, (**b**) applying forceps to a dental model

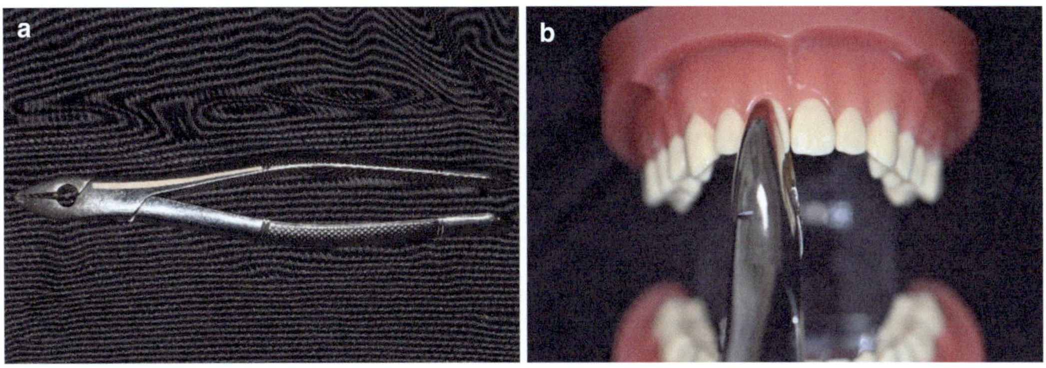


**Fig. 3.5** (**a**) Maxillary anterior forceps, (**b**) applying forceps to a dental model

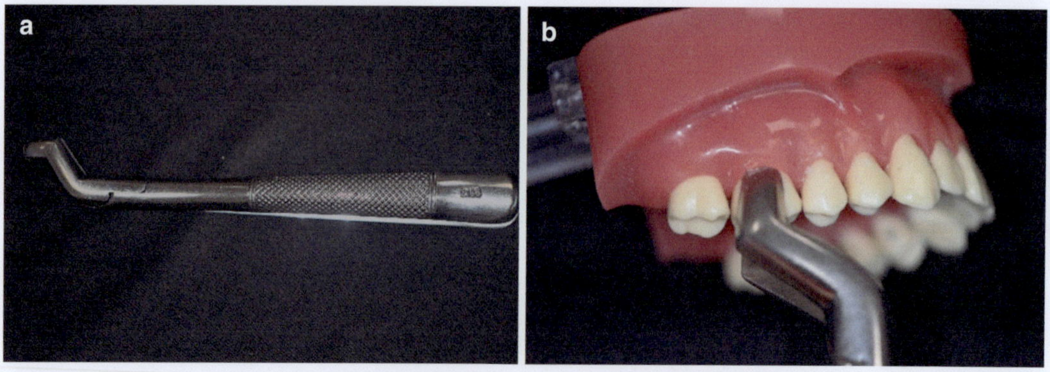

**Fig. 3.6** (**a**) Maxillary molar forceps, (**b**) applying forceps to a dental model

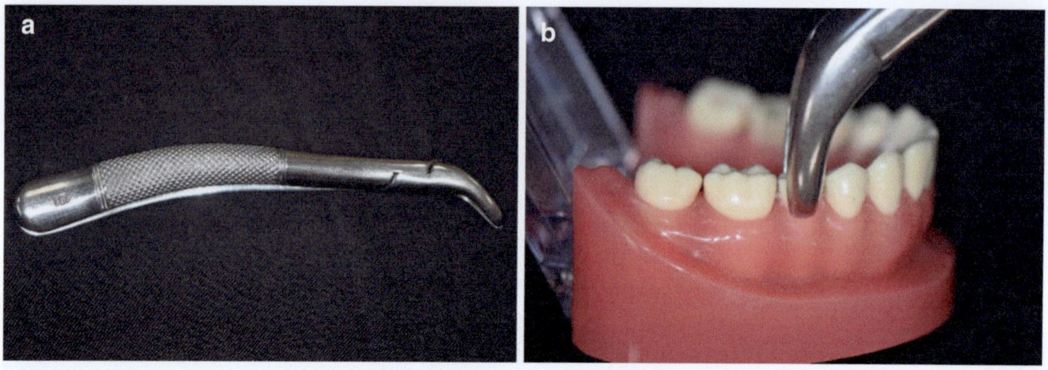

**Fig. 3.7** (**a**) Universal mandibular forceps, (**b**) applying forceps to a dental model

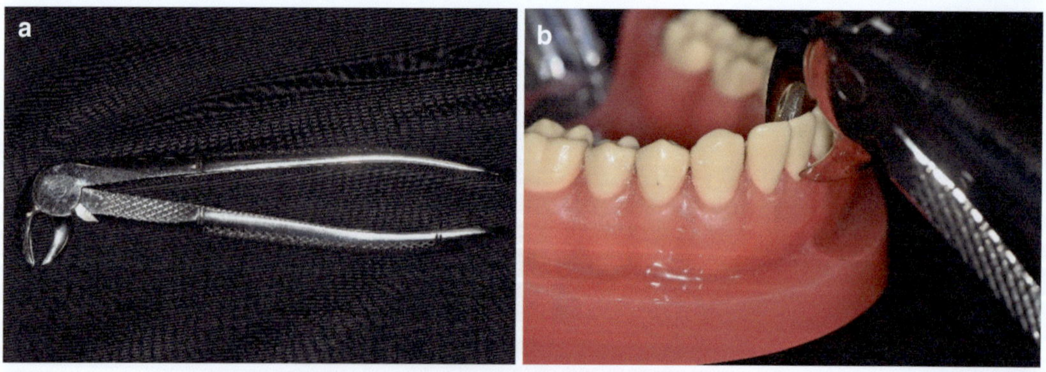

**Fig. 3.8** (**a**) Mandibular anterior forceps, (**b**) applying forceps to a dental model

– Mandibular molar forceps (No. 17 or No. 222) (Fig. 3.9.): These are specific for lower molars, designed to navigate around the tongue and lower jaw structure.
– Cowhorn forceps (No. 23): These are designed for lower molars, especially when the crowns are severely decayed or broken down. The "cowhorn" shape allows the forceps to grip the roots for more effective extraction.

• Pediatric forceps: Smaller in size, these forceps are specifically designed for

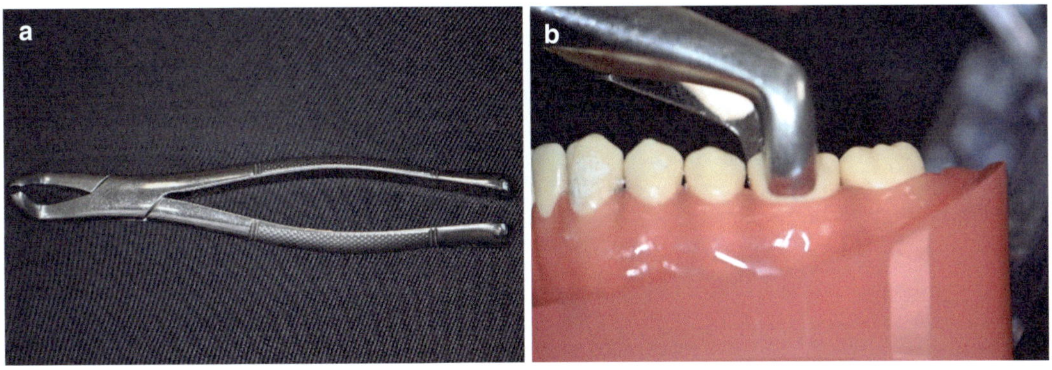


**Fig. 3.9.** (**a**) Mandibular molar forceps, (**b**) applying forceps to a dental model

extracting primary (baby) teeth. They are proportionate to the smaller teeth and jaws of children.

The choice of forceps depends on several factors, including the tooth's position, size, and condition, as well as the dentist's preference and experience. Proper selection and use of these forceps are vital for successful extractions with minimal trauma to the surrounding tissues.

2. Selection Criteria for Instruments Based on Tooth Type and Position

   The selection of the appropriate instrument is critical and depends on the type and position of the tooth.

   (a) Tooth type: The shape and size of the tooth determine the choice of instrument. Incisors and canines, with their single roots, require different forceps compared to multi-rooted molars. The curvature of the roots also plays a role; teeth with straight roots can be extracted with standard instruments, while those with curved or hooked roots may require specialized forceps or elevators.

   (b) Position in the mouth: The position of the tooth in the mouth influences the choice of instrument. For instance, teeth in the back of the mouth may be more challenging to reach and may require forceps with longer handles or specific angles.

## 3.5 Techniques for Simple Extraction

1. Step-by-Step Procedural Guide
   (a) Preparation: Ensure all necessary instruments are sterilized and ready. The patient should be in a comfortable position, and local anesthesia administered to numb the extraction area.
   (b) Initial assessment: Examine the tooth and surrounding tissues one last time to confirm the extraction plan.
   (c) Soft tissue management: If needed, use a periosteal elevator to reflect the gum tissue away from the tooth.
2. Loosening the Tooth
   (a) Using elevators: Begin by gently inserting an appropriate elevator between the tooth and the surrounding alveolar bone. Use a twisting or rocking motion to create space and disrupt the periodontal ligaments.
   (b) Gradual application of force: Increase the force gradually, being careful not to fracture the tooth or damage surrounding tissues. The goal is to expand the socket and separate the tooth from its ligament attachment.
3. Applying the Correct Force and Angle
   (a) Selecting forceps: Choose the appropriate forceps based on the tooth's location and shape. Position the beaks of the forceps firmly around the neck of the tooth.

   (b) Controlled force application: Apply a controlled force using a slow, steady, and consistent pressure. Avoid abrupt or excessive force to minimize the risk of tooth fracture or injury to the jawbone.
   (c) Correct angling: Apply force in the direction of the tooth's long axis initially, followed by gentle buccal (toward the cheek) and lingual (toward the tongue) movements to further loosen the tooth.
4. Extracting the Tooth
   (a) Final elevation: Once the tooth is sufficiently loosened, use the forceps to gently lift it out of the socket. Ensure the entire root structure is intact upon removal.
   (b) Socket inspection: Examine the socket for any remaining root fragments or bone spurs, which should be carefully removed.
5. Handling Complications During Extraction
   (a) Tooth fracture: In case of a tooth fracture, assess the situation. If the root remains, use root tip picks or elevators to gently remove it, taking care not to damage the surrounding bone.
   (b) Bleeding and infection control: Manage excessive bleeding with gauze and pressure. Prescribe antibiotics if there is a risk of infection.
6. Tips for Efficient and Safe Extraction
   (a) Atraumatic technique: Use techniques that minimize trauma to surrounding tissues, preserving bone and gum integrity for future restorative procedures or implants.
   (b) Patient communication: Keep the patient informed throughout the procedure to ease anxiety.
   (c) Continuous assessment: Be vigilant for signs of distress in the patient or complications during the procedure.
   (d) Post-extraction instructions: Provide clear post-extraction care instructions, including oral hygiene, diet, and medication.

## 3.6 Post-Extraction Care

1. Immediate Post-Extraction Instructions for Patients
   (a) Bite down on gauze: Immediately after extraction, patients should bite down gently but firmly on a gauze pad placed over the extraction site. This helps to reduce bleeding and allows a clot to form in the socket. The gauze should be kept in place for about 30 to 60 min.
   (b) Rest and activity limitation: Patients should rest for at least 24 h post-extraction and avoid any strenuous activities as they can increase blood pressure and may cause more bleeding from the extraction site.
   (c) Avoid disturbing the site: Patients should be advised not to rinse, spit forcefully, or drink from a straw for at least 24 h as these actions can dislodge the clot, leading to a painful condition known as dry socket.
2. Managing Bleeding and Pain
   (a) Control bleeding: If bleeding continues, an additional gauze pad should be placed and bitten down on for another 30 min. If heavy bleeding persists, a moistened tea bag can be used as the tannic acid helps to form a clot.
   (b) Pain management: Over-the-counter pain relievers like ibuprofen or acetaminophen can be recommended. If the pain is severe, a stronger, prescription pain medication may be prescribed.
3. Recommendations for Healing and Avoiding Complications
   (a) Oral hygiene: After 24 h, patients can gently rinse their mouth with warm salt water several times a day to reduce swelling and relieve pain. They should be careful to avoid the extraction site when brushing and flossing their other teeth.
   (b) Diet: Soft foods should be eaten for a few days post-extraction. Hot and spicy foods, as well as seeds and small grains, should

be avoided as they can get lodged in the extraction site.

(c) Avoid smoking and alcohol: Smoking should be avoided as it can impede healing, and alcohol can interfere with the effectiveness of any prescribed medication.

4. Follow-Up Procedures and Patient Education
   (a) Scheduled follow-up: A follow-up appointment may be necessary to ensure proper healing, especially in cases of complicated extractions or if sutures are placed.
   (b) Education on signs of complications: Patients should be informed about signs of complications such as excessive bleeding, severe pain, swelling, or signs of infection. They should be encouraged to contact the dental office if they experience any of these symptoms.
   (c) Long-term care: Discuss the importance of replacing the extracted tooth to prevent shifting of the remaining teeth and to maintain oral function and aesthetics. Options can include bridges, dentures, or dental implants.

## 3.7 Conclusion

In summary, the process of simple tooth extraction, though common, plays a critical role in dental practice and patient health. This procedure, necessitated by various conditions such as severe tooth decay, gum disease, or for orthodontic preparations, must be approached with a deep understanding of dental anatomy and patient-specific considerations. The text has systematically explored the techniques and principles that govern effective and safe tooth extraction, highlighting the importance of precision and patient care.

Simple extractions, while less complex than surgical extractions, require meticulous planning and execution to ensure patient comfort and to prevent complications. The discussion underscored the necessity of a thorough patient evaluation, the use of appropriate extraction instruments, and the application of proper techniques to minimize trauma to surrounding tissues. Additionally, the significance of post-extraction care to facilitate healing and maintain oral hygiene was emphasized.

This exploration into simple tooth extraction techniques aims to enhance the proficiency of dental professionals, ensuring they are equipped with the necessary knowledge and skills to perform extractions safely and effectively. In doing so, it contributes to the overarching goal of maintaining and improving oral health, underscoring the essential role of dental practitioners in patient care and well-being.

## References


1. Richards W, Ameen J, Coll AM, Higgs G. Reasons for tooth extraction in four general dental practices in South Wales. Br Dent J. 2005;198(5):275–8. https://doi.org/10.1038/sj.bdj.4812119.
2. Broers DLM, Dubois L, de Lange J, Su N, de Jongh A. Reasons for tooth removal in adults: a systematic review. Int Dent J. 2022;72(1):52–7. https://doi.org/10.1016/j.identj.2021.01.011.
3. Wilson W, Taubert KA, Gewitz M, et al. Prevention of infective endocarditis: guidelines from the American Heart Association: a guideline from the American Heart Association Rheumatic Fever, Endocarditis, and Kawasaki Disease Committee, Council on Cardiovascular Disease in the Young, and the Council on Clinical Cardiology, Council on Cardiovascular Surgery and Anesthesia, and the Quality of Care and Outcomes Research Interdisciplinary Working Group. Circulation. 2007;116(15):1736–54. https://doi.org/10.1161/CIRCULATIONAHA.106.183095.
4. Abdullah WA, Khalil H. Dental extraction in patients on warfarin treatment. Clin Cosmet Investig Dent. 2014;6:65–9. https://doi.org/10.2147/CCIDE.S68641.
5. Ruggiero SL, Dodson TB, Aghaloo T, Carlson ER, Ward BB, Kademani D. American Association of Oral and Maxillofacial Surgeons' position paper on medication-related osteonecrosis of the Jaws-2022 update. J Oral Maxillofac Surg. 2022;80(5):920–43. https://doi.org/10.1016/j.joms.2022.02.008.

# 4 Extraction of Supernumerary Teeth

## Contents



## 4.1 Introduction

The discovery and management of supernumerary teeth, particularly in the context of pediatric dentistry, is a subject of considerable clinical importance and interest. These additional teeth, often undetected until revealed through radiographic examinations during routine dental checkups or specific evaluations for the non-eruption of maxillary incisors in children, present a unique challenge to dental practitioners. The phenomenon of supernumerary teeth, while not exceedingly common, is frequent enough to merit a dedicated approach in terms of diagnosis, treatment planning, and execution.

Supernumerary teeth, or hyperdontia, manifest in various forms and locations, with a significant predilection for the anterior maxilla. The most prevalent type found in this region is known as mesiodens. These teeth can range in shape from conical to tuberculate, and in orientation from vertical to inverted, each variation presenting its own set of challenges and implications for treatment. The presence of supernumerary teeth can lead to a myriad of dental complications, including but not limited to, the delayed or impeded eruption of adjacent teeth, crowding, and the displacement or rotation of permanent teeth.

The treatment of supernumerary teeth is not a one-size-fits-all approach. It necessitates a thorough evaluation of several factors including the age of the patient, the type and position of the supernumerary tooth, its effect on adjacent teeth,


S.-G. Kim et al., *Advanced Strategies for Tooth Extraction in Dentistry*,
https://doi.org/10.1007/978-981-97-6532-4_4

and the overall dental and orthodontic treatment goals for the individual. The relationship between the supernumerary tooth and adjacent structures, particularly the roots of adjacent teeth, is of paramount importance and should be carefully assessed through appropriate radiographic techniques.

In some cases, supernumerary teeth may erupt naturally and become clinically visible, allowing for a more straightforward approach to management. However, in instances where these teeth remain impacted or only partially erupted, a more complex treatment strategy involving surgical intervention may be necessary. The surgical extraction of supernumerary teeth, particularly when ankylosed or in a complex position, requires meticulous planning and execution to avoid potential complications and to ensure the best possible outcome for the patient.

The following chapter delves into the intricacies of diagnosing and managing supernumerary and ankylosed teeth, providing a comprehensive guide for the practitioner faced with these challenges. From the initial discovery of these additional teeth through radiographic examination to the final considerations in their removal, this chapter aims to equip the reader with the knowledge and understanding necessary to navigate this complex and fascinating area of dental practice.

## 4.2 Etiology of Supernumerary Teeth

The development of supernumerary teeth is a complex phenomenon, the exact causes of which remain somewhat elusive despite numerous studies and theories. The etiology of these extra teeth is multifactorial, with several hypotheses attempting to explain their occurrence. One of the most prevalent theories suggests that supernumerary teeth result from a dichotomy of the tooth bud. This process involves the splitting or partitioning of a single tooth bud into two separate entities, leading to the formation of an additional tooth structure [1]. This theory provides a plausible explanation for the physical manifestation of these extra teeth but does not fully account for the underlying biological mechanisms.

The hyperactivity theory presents another perspective, proposing that under certain conditions, the dental lamina, a band of epithelial cells that gives rise to tooth buds, exhibits localized, independent hyperactivity [2–6]. This hyperactivity could lead to the proliferation of dental tissue and the subsequent formation of supernumerary teeth. While this theory offers insight into the potential developmental processes involved, it is still subject to ongoing research and debate.

Genetic factors undeniably play a crucial role in the development of supernumerary teeth. Studies have demonstrated a higher incidence of these teeth in children who have family members or siblings with supernumerary teeth compared to those without such a familial link [7]. This correlation strongly suggests a hereditary component, although the specific genes and mechanisms involved are yet to be fully delineated.

Recent studies have begun to shed light on the molecular aspects of supernumerary tooth formation. Genes and signaling pathways associated with tooth morphogenesis, such as Wnt, FGF, BMP, and Shh, have been implicated in the development of these extra teeth [6, 8–10]. These pathways play critical roles in the regulation of cell growth, differentiation, and patterning during embryonic development, and their dysregulation may contribute to the formation of supernumerary teeth. However, the exact molecular mechanisms remain unclear, and further research is necessary to elucidate the intricate processes involved.

In conclusion, the etiology of supernumerary teeth is a multifaceted and complex subject. While various theories provide insights into potential mechanisms, the precise cause remains unknown. Genetic predispositions combined with local environmental factors and molecular pathways likely contribute to their development. Ongoing research into the genetic and molecular basis of supernumerary teeth will be crucial in unraveling the mystery of their etiology and could potentially lead to more targeted and effective management strategies.

## 4.3 Prevalence of Supernumerary Teeth

Understanding the prevalence of supernumerary teeth is crucial for anticipating and managing these occurrences in dental practice. The frequency of these additional teeth varies significantly across different populations, dentitions, and demographic factors. In primary dentition, the prevalence of supernumerary teeth is relatively low, ranging between 0.3% and 0.8% [3, 11, 12]. However, this incidence increases in permanent dentition, with reported rates between 1.2% and 6.0% [3, 11, 12]. This suggests that the likelihood of encountering supernumerary teeth is higher in older children and adults, emphasizing the need for ongoing vigilance in radiographic examinations throughout different life stages.

Gender plays a significant role in the prevalence of supernumerary teeth in permanent dentition. Males are more frequently affected than females, with a 1.37 times higher risk of having supernumerary teeth [1]. This gender disparity highlights the need for a tailored approach in the screening and management of supernumerary teeth, particularly in male patients. Racial and ethnic differences also influence the prevalence of these extra teeth. Studies have shown that Asian populations exhibit a higher prevalence of supernumerary teeth compared to Caucasian populations [13, 14]. This variation underscores the importance of considering racial and ethnic backgrounds when assessing the risk and prevalence of supernumerary teeth in different patient populations.

Supernumerary teeth can manifest in various forms, including single or multiple, unilateral or bilateral, erupted or impacted, and in either jaw. While the occurrence of a single supernumerary tooth is more common, multiple supernumerary teeth are typically associated with syndromes or other disorders. Conditions commonly associated with multiple supernumerary teeth include cleft lip and palate, cleidocranial dysplasia, Down's syndrome, and Gardner syndrome [2, 3, 15–17]. In patients with cleft lip and palate, the prevalence of supernumerary teeth is notable, particularly on the affected side of the cleft. Studies have reported an incidence rate of 22.2% for supernumerary teeth in these cases [18]. This increased prevalence is often attributed to the fragmentation of the dental lamina during cleft formation, leading to the development of extra tooth structures.

Cleidocranial dysplasia presents another condition with a significant association with supernumerary teeth. In this disorder, the prevalence of supernumerary teeth in the anterior maxilla is 22%, while in the molar region, it is 5% [19]. This highlights the variability in the location and prevalence of supernumerary teeth even within specific syndromic contexts.

Interestingly, the prevalence of supernumerary teeth does not vary by gender in primary dentition. However, in permanent dentition, it is about twice as high in males as in females. This difference further illustrates the complex interplay of genetic, developmental, and possibly hormonal factors in the manifestation of supernumerary teeth. The prevalence of supernumerary teeth is influenced by a multitude of factors, including dentition type, gender, race, and associated syndromes or conditions. Understanding these variables is crucial for dental professionals in predicting, diagnosing, and managing supernumerary teeth effectively in diverse patient populations.

## 4.4 Classification of Supernumerary Teeth

Supernumerary teeth are classified based on their morphology and location. In primary dentition, they may appear normal or conical. In permanent dentition, they exhibit a wide range of morphologies and are broadly categorized into conical, tuberculate, supplemental, and odontoma types (Fig. 4.1).

1. Conical

   This type is peg-shaped and most common in permanent dentition. Conical supernumerary teeth often lead to rotation or displacement of permanent incisors [20].

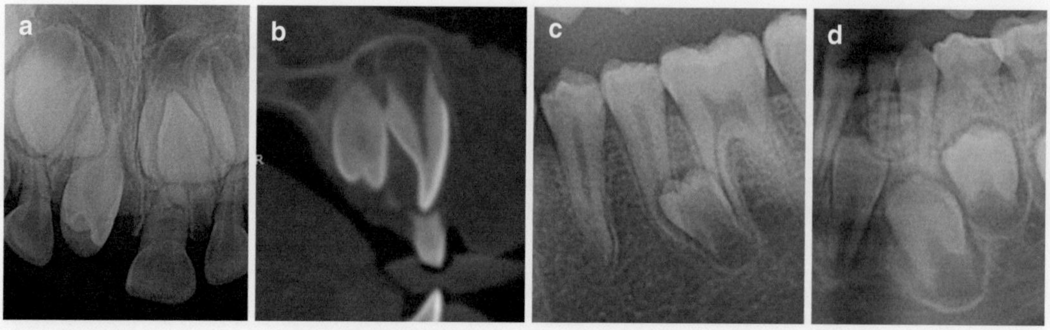


**Fig. 4.1** Classification of supernumerary tooth. (**a**) Conical, (**b**) tuberculate, (**c**) supplemental, (**d**) odontoma

2. Tuberculate

   Characterized by one or more cusps or tubercles, often described as barrel-shaped or inverted. Root formation is usually delayed compared to permanent incisors. They often appear in pairs and are usually located palatally to permanent incisors. Eruption delays are not common, but they can cause delayed eruption of permanent incisors [21].
3. Supplemental

   These resemble normal teeth and are additional in number. Most commonly, they duplicate the maxillary lateral incisors, occasionally seen in premolars or molars. They predominantly occur in primary dentition and rarely become impacted [22].
4. Odontoma

   Some classify odontomas as a type of supernumerary tooth, although they are generally categorized as odontogenic tumors. There are two forms: composite odontoma, which retains a toothlike structure, and complex odontoma, presenting as a diffuse mass of dental tissue [23].

## 4.5 Clinical Problems Associated with Supernumerary Teeth

Supernumerary teeth, while fascinating in their occurrence, can lead to a range of clinical problems (Fig. 4.2). These issues vary in complexity and impact, affecting not only the dentition but also the broader treatment plans for affected individuals. Understanding these complications is crucial for effective management and treatment planning.

1. Eruption Delay

   The presence of supernumerary teeth is a well-documented cause of eruption failure, particularly for maxillary incisors. These extra teeth can lead to the retention of primary teeth and subsequent issues in the eruption of permanent lateral incisors [24]. The delay or failure in eruption due to supernumerary teeth is not limited to the anterior maxilla; supernumerary teeth in other locations can also adversely affect the eruption of adjacent teeth. These delays can lead to significant treatment challenges and may require early intervention to prevent long-term complications.
2. Displacement of Tooth Position

   Supernumerary teeth frequently cause the displacement of permanent teeth, with varying degrees of severity. The most common manifestation of this is the crown displacement of incisors, often observed in children experiencing eruption delays [25]. This displacement can lead to aesthetic concerns, functional problems, and the need for complex orthodontic treatment to correct the tooth alignment.
3. Complications in Cleft Lip and Palate Patients

   In individuals with cleft lip and palate, supernumerary teeth can significantly complicate bone grafting procedures. If these teeth have erupted, it is generally recommended to extract them first, allowing complete healing of the extraction site before proceeding with

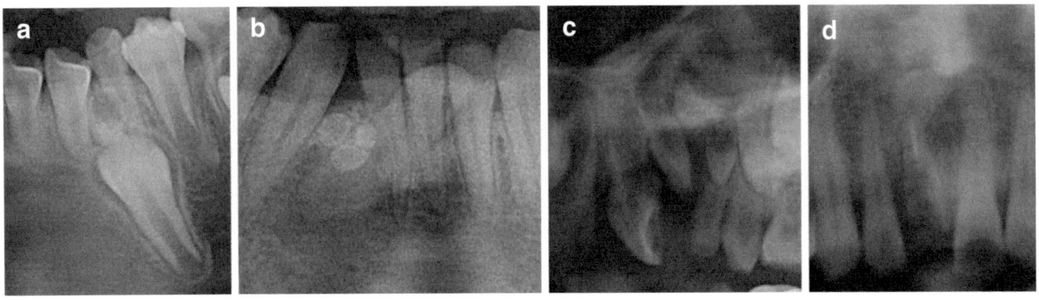


**Fig. 4.2** Clinical problems associated with supernumerary tooth. (**a**) Eruption delay, (**b**) tooth displacement, (**c**) problem in cleft lip and palate, (**d**) implant placement obstruction

bone grafting. For impacted supernumerary teeth, simultaneous extraction during bone grafting is often advised. However, due to the variety of presentations in cleft lip and palate patients, consultation with a specialized cleft team is essential before proceeding with extraction [26].

4. Implant Placement Obstruction

   In cases where dental implants are planned, impacted supernumerary teeth can obstruct the implant sites. These teeth need to be extracted prior to implant placement, and in some cases, bone grafting might be required to ensure adequate support for the implant. The presence of supernumerary teeth at potential implant sites necessitates careful planning and consideration of the timing and sequence of surgical interventions.

5. Asymptomatic Supernumerary Teeth

   Not all supernumerary teeth cause immediate clinical problems. Some remain asymptomatic, not causing issues such as delayed eruption, crowding, or cyst formation, and are only detected incidentally during radiographic examinations. In such cases, extraction may not be immediately necessary. However, patients should be informed about the potential for future complications, such as ankylosis or cyst formation, and the need for regular monitoring to ensure that any changes in the status of these teeth are promptly addressed.

In summary, the presence of supernumerary teeth can lead to a variety of clinical problems, from eruption delays and tooth displacement to complications in specialized surgical procedures. The management of these issues requires a comprehensive understanding of the potential complications, careful assessment and monitoring of the affected individuals, and a tailored approach to treatment that considers the unique needs and circumstances of each patient.

## 4.6 Treatment of Supernumerary Teeth

The treatment of supernumerary teeth is a multifaceted and individualized process, considering various factors such as the type and location of the supernumerary tooth, potential implant placement, and specific considerations in patients with conditions like cleft lip and palate. Treatment options generally include extraction, observation without extraction, and specific management strategies following extraction.

1. Extraction Indications

   Extraction is typically recommended in several scenarios. These include cases where supernumerary teeth cause delayed or obstructed eruption of maxillary permanent incisors, displacement of adjacent teeth, or are associated with pathological conditions like cysts. Additionally, extraction is advised when supernumerary teeth interfere with orthodontic tooth movement, obstruct bone grafting procedures in cleft lip and palate patients, are present at future implant sites, or are erupted supernumerary teeth causing aesthetic or

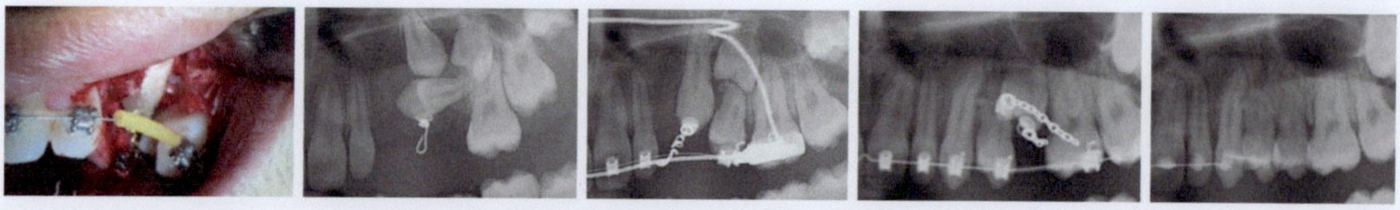

**Fig. 4.3** Surgically forced eruption of permanent tooth (#23,24,25) (by Courtesy of prof. Kim SH)

functional issues. The decision to extract is based on a careful assessment of the potential benefits and risks, considering the individual's overall dental health and treatment goals.

2. Observation Without Extraction

   In certain cases, supernumerary teeth may not necessitate immediate extraction. This approach is indicated for supernumerary teeth that do not affect the eruption of adjacent teeth, where no orthodontic treatment is necessary or planned, are not associated with pathological conditions, or when the extraction poses a clear risk of damaging adjacent structures. Observation without extraction requires regular monitoring to ensure that the supernumerary teeth do not begin to cause problems over time.

3. Post-Extraction Management of Impacted Permanent Teeth

   Following the extraction of supernumerary teeth, the impacted permanent teeth often proceed to erupt normally. Raji Pescia reported that about 65.5% of impacted teeth erupt normally within 18 months post-extraction [26]. However, this is not always the case, and some practitioners recommend forced eruption post-extraction to facilitate the process. Witsenburg and Boering noted that only 54% of mandibular permanent teeth erupt naturally post-extraction of supernumerary teeth, hence the recommendation for forced eruption using a gold chain or other orthodontic devices. The treatment plan for post-extraction management should consider factors like the root formation of the impacted permanent tooth, the patient's age, and the specific location of the tooth in the maxilla or mandible [15] (Fig. 4.3).

In summary, the treatment of supernumerary teeth is a tailored process that must consider the individual patient's needs, the specific characteristics of the supernumerary teeth, and the potential impact on adjacent structures and future dental treatments. Whether through extraction, observation, or specific post-extraction management, the goal is to ensure the best possible outcome for the patient's oral health and overall well-being.

## 4.7 Extraction Techniques

1. Mesiodens Extraction

   The extraction of mesiodens, a type of supernumerary tooth commonly found in the anterior maxilla, requires precise planning and execution. Prior to extraction, a thorough radiographic examination is indispensable to accurately determine the supernumerary tooth's position relative to the normal teeth and critical anatomical structures.

   (a) Pre-extraction Radiographic Examination

   Standard panoramic radiographs often fall short in providing the necessary detail to discern whether the supernumerary tooth is located labially or palatally. Cone-beam CT imaging is recommended due to its superior ability to delineate the precise location and orientation of the mesiodens. As an alternative, standard radiographs taken from two different horizontal angles can be utilized to ascertain the tooth's position relative to the roots of normal teeth. The information gathered from these imaging techniques informs the surgical approach and helps mitigate the risk of complications.

   (b) Extraction Technique for Palatally Located Mesiodens

   When the mesiodens is located on the palatal side, a crestal incision is typically employed for access and extraction.

Surgeons must exercise caution to avoid damage to the incisive nerve and permanent teeth. Following the extraction, it is imperative to completely remove the surrounding follicular sac to prevent potential cyst formation or recurrence. Achieving adequate hemostasis and closing the surgical site with absorbable 4-0 sutures ensure proper healing and reduces the risk of postoperative complications (Fig. 4.4).

(c) Extraction Technique for Labially Located Mesiodens

For mesiodens located on the labial side, a vestibular incision is preferred. The Partsch method can also be employed, which involves creating a mucoperiosteal flap at the gingival margin. This approach is favored for labially located mesiodens, especially in the anterior maxilla, due to aesthetic considerations. Minimizing visible scarring and preserving the gingival architecture are crucial in these areas, given their visibility and impact on the patient's smile and overall appearance.

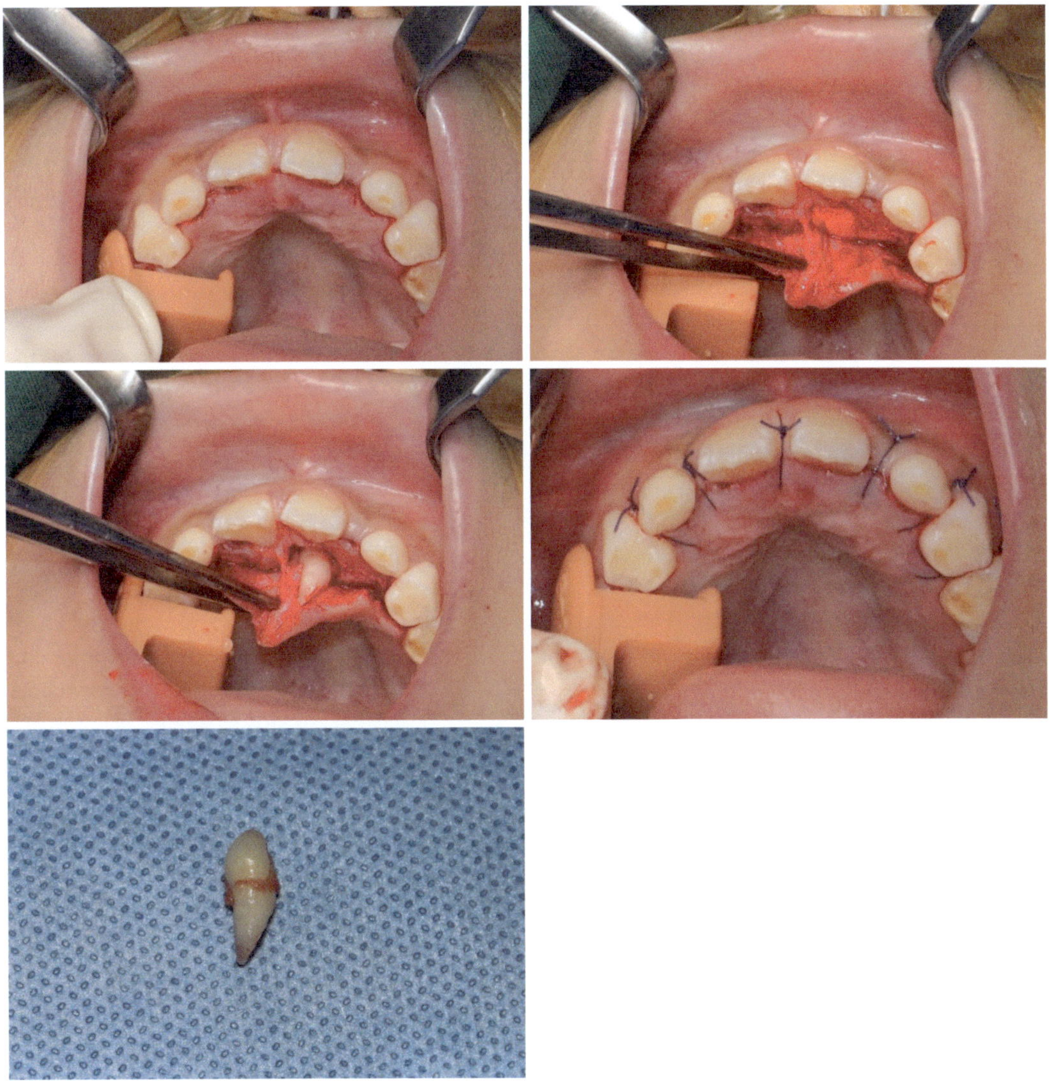

**Fig. 4.4** Mesiodens extraction

In summary, the extraction of mesiodens requires a nuanced approach tailored to its position—whether palatally or labially located. The choice of surgical technique, whether a crestal incision for palatally located mesiodens or a vestibular approach for labially located ones, is determined based on detailed pre-extraction radiographic assessment. Careful surgical execution, coupled with meticulous attention to the removal of the follicular sac and proper wound closure, is essential for successful outcomes and patient satisfaction.

2. Extraction of Ankylosed Teeth

   Ankylosed teeth present a unique challenge in dental extractions due to the fusion of the tooth root to the surrounding bone. Understanding the nature of the ankylosis and the appropriate techniques for extraction is crucial for successful outcomes and minimizing complications.

   (a) Types of Ankylosis

      Most ankylosed teeth exhibit fibrous ankylosis, where the root is fused to the bone through a fibrous connection rather than direct bony contact. This type of ankylosis often allows for slightly easier extraction, as the fibrous tissue can sometimes be separated. True bony ankylosis, however, is more challenging. In these rare cases, the root and alveolar bone are indistinguishable, creating a solid union that is difficult to disrupt. The alveolar bone often becomes significantly dense around the ankylosed tooth, further complicating the extraction process.

   (b) Extraction Techniques

      Given the complexities associated with ankylosed teeth, certain specialized techniques are usually preferred. Root division or odontotomy is often the method of choice. This involves sectioning the tooth into smaller parts to facilitate a more manageable and less traumatic removal. By dividing the tooth, the dentist can minimize the force needed to extract each piece, reducing the risk of damaging surrounding bone and tissues (Fig. 4.5).

   (c) Post-Extraction Care

      Due to the increased density of the alveolar bone and the potential for significant trauma during extraction, meticulous care is essential following the removal of an ankylosed tooth. Suturing the extraction wound is highly recommended to promote healing, minimize the risk of infection, and prevent complications such as osteomyelitis. This is particularly important in cases of bony ankylosis, where the bone's integrity may be compromised.

   The extraction of ankylosed teeth requires a strategic approach that accounts for the nature of the ankylosis and the condition of the surrounding bone. Understanding whether the ankylosis is fibrous or bony guides the choice of extraction technique, with root division or odontotomy being preferred methods. Ensuring proper post-extraction care, including suturing the wound, is crucial to prevent complications and promote healing. With careful planning and execution, the challenges posed by ankylosed teeth can be effectively managed.

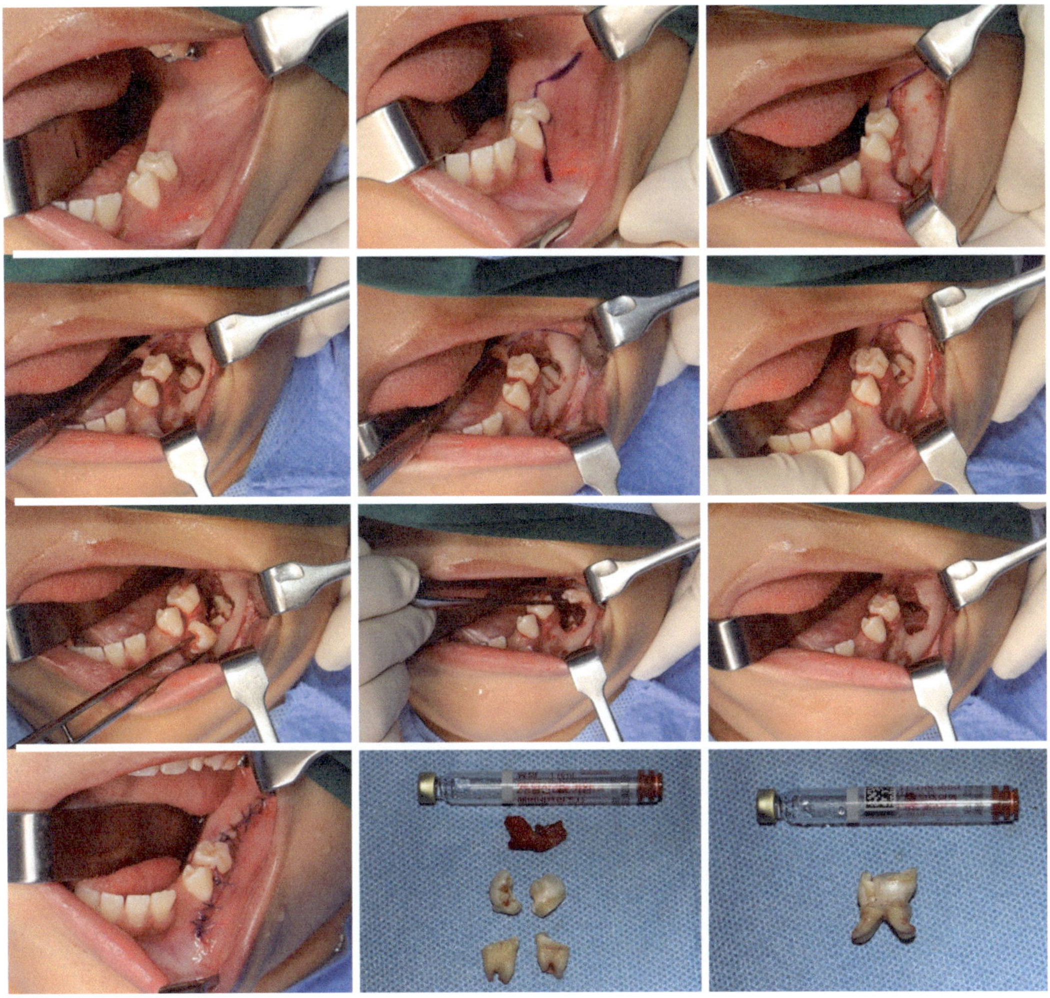

**Fig. 4.5** Extraction of ankylosed tooth

## 4.8 Conclusion

This chapter provides an extensive overview of supernumerary teeth, their clinical implications, and management strategies, serving as an invaluable resource for dental professionals seeking a thorough understanding of this complex topic.

## References

1. Anthonappa RP, King NM, Rabie ABM. Aetiology of supernumerary teeth: a literature review. Eur Arch Paediatr Dent. 2013;14:279–88. https://doi.org/10.1007/s40368-013-0082-z.
2. Ferrés-Padró E, Prats-Armengol J, Ferrés-Amat E. A descriptive study of 113 unerupted supernumerary teeth in 79 pediatric patients in Barcelona. Med Oral Patol Oral Cir Bucal. 2009;14:E146–52. http://www.medicinaoral.com/medoralfree01/v14i3/medoralv14i3p146.pdf
3. Rajab LD, Hamdan MAM. Supernumerary teeth: review of the literature and a survey of 152 cases. Int J Paediatr Dent. 2002;12:244–54. https://doi.org/10.1046/j.1365-263X.2002.00366.x.
4. Ata-Ali F, Ata-Ali J, Peñarrocha-Oltra D, Peñarrocha-Diago M. Prevalence, etiology, diagnosis, treatment and complications of supernumerary teeth. J Clin Exp Dent. 2014;6:e414–8. https://doi.org/10.4317/jced.51499.
5. De Oliveira Gomes C, Drummond SN, Jham BC, Abdo EN, Mesquita RA. A survey of 460 supernumerary teeth in Brazilian children and adolescents. Int J Paediatr Dent. 2008;18:98–106. https://doi.org/10.1111/j.1365-263X.2007.00862.x.

6. Fleming PS, Xavier GM, DiBiase AT, Cobourne MT. Revisiting the supernumerary: the epidemiological and molecular basis of extra teeth. Br Dent J. 2010;208:25–30. https://doi.org/10.1038/sj.bdj.2009.1177.
7. Russell KA, Folwarczna MA. Mesiodens-diagnosis and management of a common supernumerary tooth. J Can Dent Assoc. 2003;69(6):362–6. https://www.cda-adc.ca/jcda/vol-69/issue-6/vol69_issue6.pdf#page=22
8. Lu X, Yu F, Liu J, et al. The epidemiology of supernumerary teeth and the associated molecular mechanism. Organogenesis. 2017;13:71–82. https://doi.org/10.1080/15476278.2017.1332554.
9. Adisornkanj P, Chanprasit R, Eliason S, et al. Genetic variants in protein tyrosine phosphatase non-receptor type 23 are responsible for mesiodens formation. Biology. 2023;12:393. https://doi.org/10.3390/biology12030393.
10. Küchler EC, Reis CLB, Silva-Sousa AC, et al. Exploring the association between genetic polymorphisms in genes involved in craniofacial development and isolated tooth agenesis. Front Physiol. 2021;12:723105. https://doi.org/10.3389/fphys.2021.723105.
11. Syriac G, Joseph E, Rupesh S, Philip J, Cherian SA, Mathew J. Prevalence, characteristics, and complications of supernumerary teeth in nonsyndromic pediatric population of South India: a clinical and radiographic study. J Pharm Bioallied Sci. 2017;9:S231–6. https://doi.org/10.4103/jpbs.JPBS_154_17.
12. Brook AH. Dental anomalies of number, form and size: their prevalence in British schoolchildren. J Int Assoc Dent Child. 1974;5(2):37–53.
13. Moore SR, Wilson DF, Kibble J. Sequential development of multiple supernumerary teeth in the mandibular premolar region -- a radiographic case report. Int J Paediatr Dent. 2002;12:143–5. https://doi.org/10.1046/j.1365-263X.2002.00336.x.
14. Cheng FC, Chen MH, Liu BL, et al. Nonsyndromic supernumerary teeth in patients in National Taiwan University Children's hospital. J Dent Sci. 2022;17:1612–8. https://doi.org/10.1016/j.jds.2022.07.015.
15. Cammarata-Scalisi F, Avendaño A, Callea M. Main genetic entities associated with supernumerary teeth. Arch Argent Pediatr. 2018;116:437–44. https://doi.org/10.5546/aap.2018.eng.437.
16. Shah A, Gill DS, Tredwin C, Naini FB. Diagnosis and management of supernumerary teeth. Dent Update. 2008;35:510–2, 514–6, 519–20. https://doi.org/10.12968/denu.2008.35.8.510.
17. Brook AH. A unifying aetiological explanation for anomalies of human tooth number and size. Arch Oral Biol. 1984;29:373–8. https://doi.org/10.1016/0003-9969(84)90163-8.
18. Gomes RR. Supernumerary teeth in cleft lip and palate patients. Cleft Palate Craniofac J. 2003;40(5):556–8. https://doi.org/10.1016/j.jdent.2016.03.010.
19. Jensen BL, Kreiborg S. Development of the dentition in cleidocranial dysplasia. J Oral Pathol Med. 1992;21(1):45–52. https://onlinelibrary.wiley.com/doi/pdf/10.1111/j.1600-0714.1990.tb00803.x?casa_token=KxoligNQ5wIAAAAA:LmuD1eouWtVIoNPCgKlfwUtdTeMd4F6CgU0eZc8Yt8X6cB2Ts2NU33rKMxw_Xn8AoIY1xb8Ixqkb_Vs
20. Primosch RE. Anterior supernumerary teeth—assessment and surgical intervention in children. Pediatr Dent. 1988;10(3):209–15. https://www.aapd.org/globalassets/media/publications/archives/primosch-03-02.pdf
21. Subramaniam P, Babu KLG. Prevalence of supernumerary teeth in deciduous and mixed dentition. J Indian Soc Pedod Prev Dent. 2007;25(2):73–5. https://europepmc.org/article/med/12885009
22. Garvey MT, Barry HJ, Blake M. Supernumerary teeth—an overview of classification, diagnosis and management. J Can Dent Assoc. 1999;65(11):612–6. https://www.cda-adc.ca/jcda/vol-65/issue-11/612.pdf
23. Yague-Garcia J, Berini-Aytes L. Multiple supernumerary teeth not associated with complex syndromes: a retrospective study. Med Oral Patol Oral Cir Bucal. 2009;14(7):E331–6. https://dialnet.unirioja.es/servlet/articulo?codigo=6009782
24. Gregg TA, Kinirons MJ. The effect of the position and orientation of unerupted premaxillary supernumerary teeth on eruption and displacement of permanent incisors. Int J Paediatr Dent. 1991;1(1):3–7. https://doi.org/10.1111/j.1365-263x.1991.tb00314.x.
25. Witsenburg B, Boering G. Eruption of impacted permanent upper incisors after removal of supernumerary teeth. Int J Oral Surg. 1983;12(6):423–31. https://doi.org/10.1016/S0300-9785(81)80079-8.
26. Pescia R, Kiliaridis S, Antonarakis GS. Spontaneous eruption of impacted maxillary incisors after surgical extraction of supernumerary teeth: a systematic review and meta-analysis. Clin Oral Investig. 2020;24(11):3749–59. https://doi.org/10.1007/s00784-020-03369-3.

# 5 Techniques for Managing Impacted Canine

## Contents



## 5.1 Introduction

Canines are not just fundamental to the mechanics of biting and chewing but also hold significant value in facial aesthetics. The phenomenon of canine impaction is a dental predicament where the root of the permanent tooth is entirely developed, yet it fails to erupt in alignment with the dental arch [1]. This condition, particularly concerning the maxillary canines, is not as rare as one might assume. With a reported prevalence of 1.7–4.7%, maxillary canine impaction stands as the second most common impaction after the third molars [2, 3].

The etiology behind maxillary canine impaction is multifaceted. Often, it is attributed to the delayed eruption sequence, where the eruption of the premolars precedes that of the canines. This phenomenon can be exacerbated by several factors, including the positioning of adjacent teeth, discrepancies in arch length, and disproportionate tooth size [4, 5]. Contrarily, palatal impaction of maxillary canines leans more toward a genetic predisposition. On the other hand, mandibular canine impaction, while less frequent, typically ensues post the impaction of the third molars in the mandible. The primary culprits for this are believed to be an abnormal positioning of the tooth bud, along with the potential lack of arch space and an oversized canine crown [6, 7].

Addressing impacted canines is a multifaceted process that necessitates a tailored approach for everyone. The management spectrum ranges from early interceptive strategies to more invasive surgical interventions. For cases with an anticipated permanent canine impaction, an early interceptive approach is recommended. This involves the extraction of the primary canine to make way for the permanent one, supplemented by orthodontic treatments such as rapid maxillary expansion and headgear usage. These interventions aim to create sufficient space and


S.-G. Kim et al., *Advanced Strategies for Tooth Extraction in Dentistry*,
https://doi.org/10.1007/978-981-97-6532-4_5

foster the normal eruption of the permanent canine.

For more stubborn cases, surgical exposure is a viable option. This technique entails the elevation of a gingival flap to expose the impacted canine. Subsequently, an orthodontic button is attached to the crown, and a gold chain is employed to gradually pull the tooth into its rightful position through forced eruption. In scenarios where neither interceptive nor surgical methods are viable or preferred, alternatives like artificial transplantation or extraction of the impacted canine are considered [8]. Understanding the complexity of impacted canines and the nuances of their management is crucial for dental practitioners. This chapter aims to dissect these techniques, offering insight into their methodologies, applicabilities, and potential outcomes. The goal is to enhance the clinician's ability to effectively manage this common yet challenging dental condition.

## 5.2 Extraction of Impacted Canine

1. Extraction Technique of Impacted Maxillary Canine

   In certain clinical scenarios, the natural eruption of an impacted maxillary canine is deemed highly unlikely, particularly when the space designated for the canine has closed, rendering orthodontic space creation both time-intensive and financially burdensome. In these instances, extraction of the impacted canine may be considered a more feasible option to maintain the current occlusion (Fig. 5.1). However, this decision should always be made in consultation with the patient and their guardians, ensuring a thorough understanding of the procedure's implications. Moreover, the presence or potential development of a cyst around the crown of the impacted canine further necessitates its extraction.

2. Surgical Procedure

   (a) Incision: The choice of incision—sulcular, vestibular, or mucogingival junction—is contingent upon the location of the impacted canine. For palatally impacted canines, a palatal approach may be required. The incision, typically 1–2 cm in length, should be ample to reveal the crown of the tooth fully.

   (b) Flap elevation: A full-thickness flap elevation is performed to provide a clear view of the impacted tooth and surrounding bone. Achieving adequate hemostasis during this step is crucial to minimize bleeding and improve visibility.

   (c) Bone grinding or removal: In many cases, the labial bone covering the crown of the canine is either perforated or presents as a thin film. Here, bone curettes are effective for removal. However, if the bone is significantly thicker, drilling may be necessary to access the crown.

   (d) Odontomy: This step is generally not required for children. However, adults with impacted canines often present with ankylosis, necessitating the division of the tooth. A high-speed bur is used at the cervix of the tooth to perform odontomy, facilitating easier extraction.

   (e) Extraction using elevator: An extraction elevator is employed to separately remove the crown and the root of the tooth. This method ensures a more controlled and precise removal, especially in complex cases.

   (f) Hemostasis: Post-surgical bleeding can lead to swelling and bruising, which are common concerns for many patients. Effective hemostasis is essential to prevent these complications and ensure a smoother recovery.

   (g) Closure: The choice of suture material varies with the patient's age. In children, absorbable 4-0 vicryl is preferred for continuous suturing, which negates the need for stitch removal. Conversely, adults may require suturing with materials like silk or nylon for optimal healing.

The extraction of impacted maxillary canines is a complex procedure that requires a meticu-

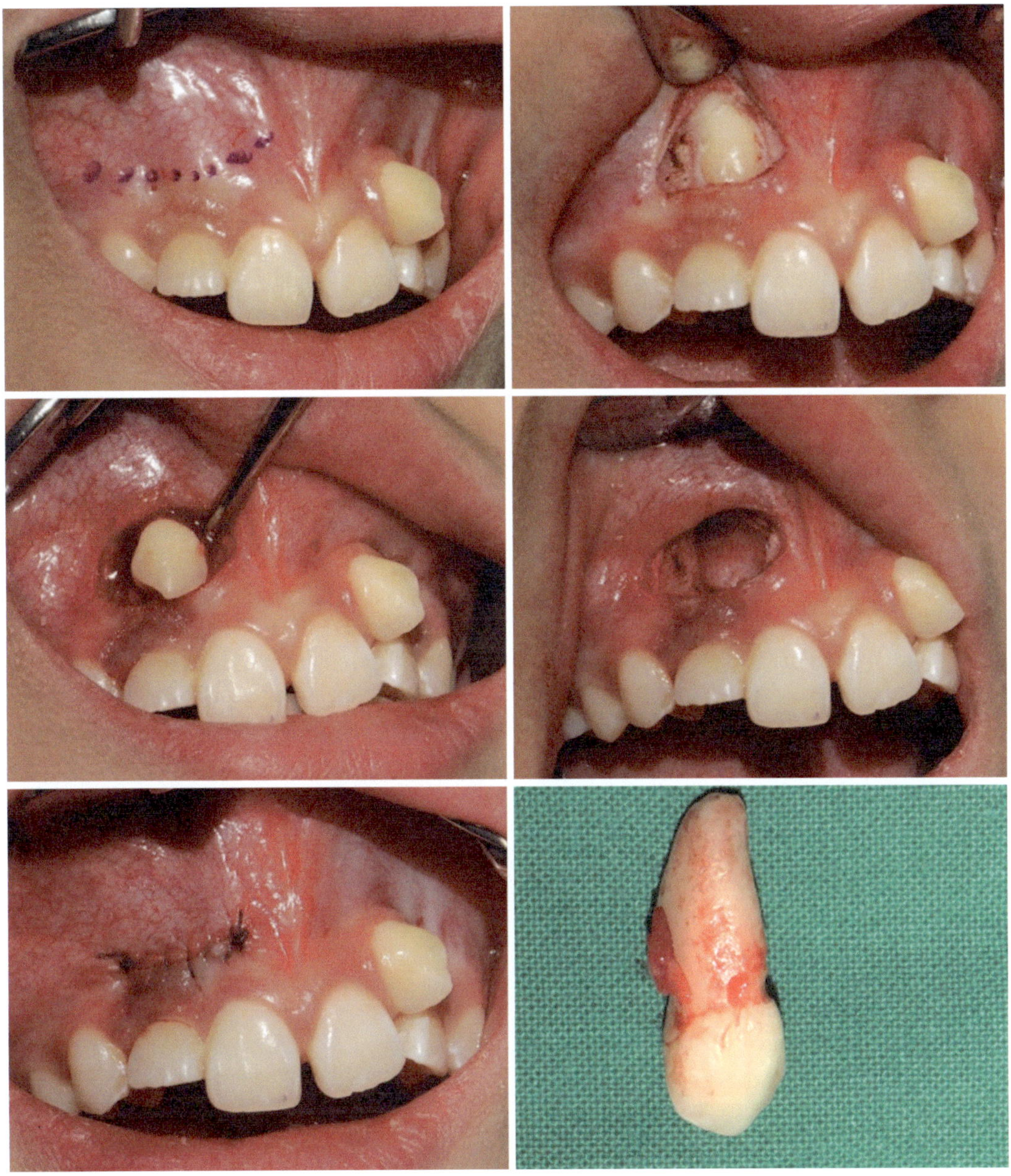

**Fig. 5.1** Extraction of impacted maxillary canine

lous approach and should be considered when other orthodontic interventions are deemed impractical or unfeasible. The technique involves several critical steps, each requiring careful execution to ensure the patient's safety and the procedure's success. As with all dental procedures, informed consent and a comprehensive understanding of the patient's medical history are paramount. This technique offers a viable alternative to traditional orthodontic interventions, providing relief and a path forward for patients with impacted canines.

## 5.3 Observation Without Extraction

In certain clinical circumstances where the space designated for an impacted canine has been occluded by the eruption of permanent premolars, and the overall maxillary and mandibular occlusion appears normal, opting for a conservative approach by simply monitoring the condition may be considered appropriate. This noninvasive strategy is contingent upon a comprehensive evaluation of the patient's dental health and a balanced risk-benefit analysis.

1. Communicating with Patients and Guardians
   (a) Informed decision-making: Central to adopting a watchful waiting strategy is the thorough communication with the patient or their guardians. They must be fully apprised of the condition, its potential progression, and the implications of choosing observation over immediate extraction.
   (b) Potential risks: It is imperative to discuss the possibility of cyst formation or inflammation around the impacted canine. While these risks might not necessitate immediate action, understanding them is crucial for future monitoring and decision-making.
   (c) Implications for future dental procedures: The presence of an impacted canine can complicate future dental interventions. For instance, if the tooth above the impacted canine is lost and implant placement is required, the impacted canine might present challenges. Discussing these scenarios helps in planning future dental care and setting realistic expectations.
2. Monitoring Strategy
   (a) Regular checkups: A structured schedule for dental checkups is crucial to monitor the status of the impacted canine. These visits allow for timely detection of any changes or developments that might necessitate intervention.
   (b) Imaging and diagnostics: Periodic imaging, such as X-rays or CT scans, may be employed to keep a close watch on the position of the impacted canine and the health of surrounding tissues.
   (c) Assessing changes in condition: Any signs of cyst formation, inflammation, or shifts in the position of the impacted canine should be meticulously recorded and assessed. Changes in the patient's symptoms or discomfort levels should also be noted.
3. Decision-making Over Time
   (a) Reevaluation: The decision to continue with observation should be regularly reevaluated based on the latest clinical findings and the patient's comfort and preferences.
   (b) Flexibility in approach: While the initial decision might be to observe, it is essential to remain open to changing the course of action if the patient's condition evolves or if potential risks start to outweigh the benefits.

Opting for a strategy of observation without immediate extraction for impacted canines is a viable route in specific clinical scenarios. However, it necessitates a comprehensive understanding of the condition, clear communication with the patient or their guardians, and a commitment to regular monitoring. This approach allows for a balanced consideration of the patient's current and future dental health, providing a foundation for informed and adaptive decision-making.

## 5.4 Forced Eruption of Impacted Teeth

1. Surgical exposure for forced eruption of impacted maxillary canine
   (a) Incision: Typically, incisions such as sulcular, vestibular, and mucogingival junction incisions can be used, and the choice depends on the location of the impacted canine. In cases where the canine is palatally impacted, a palatal approach may be

inevitable. The incision size should be about 1–2 cm, sufficient to expose the crown of the tooth (Fig. 5.2a).

(b) Flap elevation: A full-thickness flap elevation should be performed, followed by ensuring adequate hemostasis (Fig. 5.2b).

(c) Bone grinding or removal of labial bone of canine crown: In most cases of impacted canines, the labial bone over the crown is either perforated or remains as a thin film. In such cases, bone curettes can be used to remove it, or if the remaining bone is thick, a drill may be utilized for removal (Fig. 5.2c, d).

(d) Bonding of orthodontic button: Before attaching the orthodontic button, it is crucial to ensure thorough hemostasis and use dry gauze to make the canine crown completely dry. After achieving a perfectly dry state, an orthodontic resin bond is used to attach the orthodontic button (Fig. 5.2e). The placement of the button is critical for the application of orthodontic force, so its position should be carefully evaluated and selected. Generally, the button is attached to the labial surface of the canine. After the button is attached, a gold chain is connected and brought out into the oral cavity. The point where the chain is pulled out should be chosen based on what is most advantageous for applying force, either at the crestal incision site or through attached mucosa. To minimize patient discomfort, the gold chain is temporarily fixed to the crown of an adjacent tooth.

(e) Hemostasis: Many patients experience swelling and bruising due to bleeding post-surgery. Adequate hemostasis is essential to prevent these complications.

(f) Closure: In children, absorbable 4-0 vicryl can be used for continuous suturing, eliminating the need for stitch removal. In adults, suturing can be done using silk or nylon (Fig. 5.2f).

2. Clinical case of forced eruption of bilaterally impacted maxillary canines

A 9-year and 4-month-old female patient presented with bilateral maxillary canine impaction. Following the surgical exposure of both impacted maxillary canines, a forced eruption procedure was performed (Fig. 5.3).

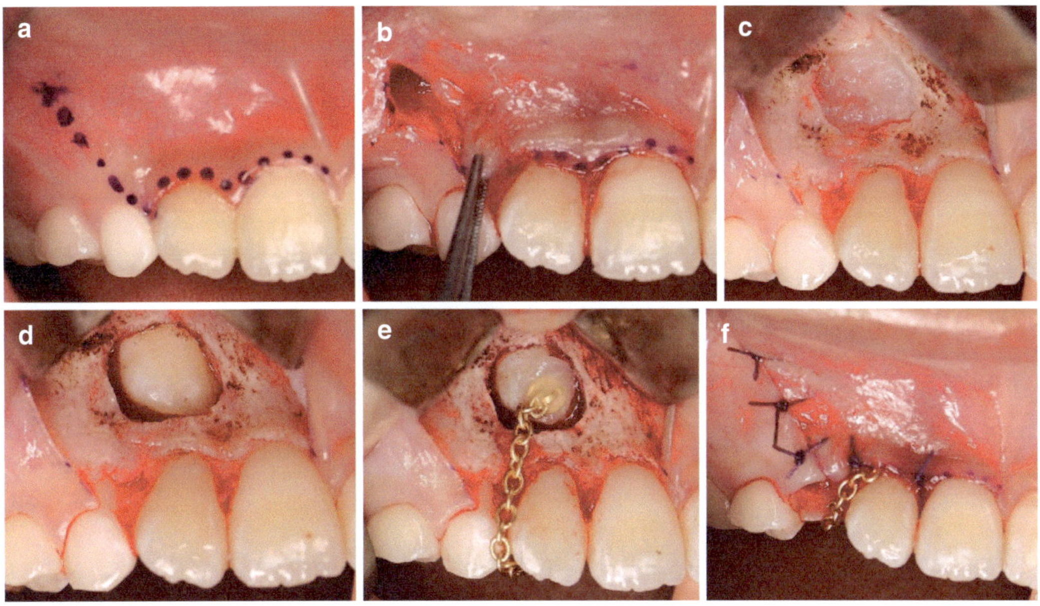


**Fig. 5.2** Surgical exposure for forced eruption of impacted maxillary canine. (**a**) Incision design, (**b**) incision and flap elevation, (**c**) exposing the canine, (**d**) removal of labial bone of canine, (**e**) bonding of button, (**f**) closure

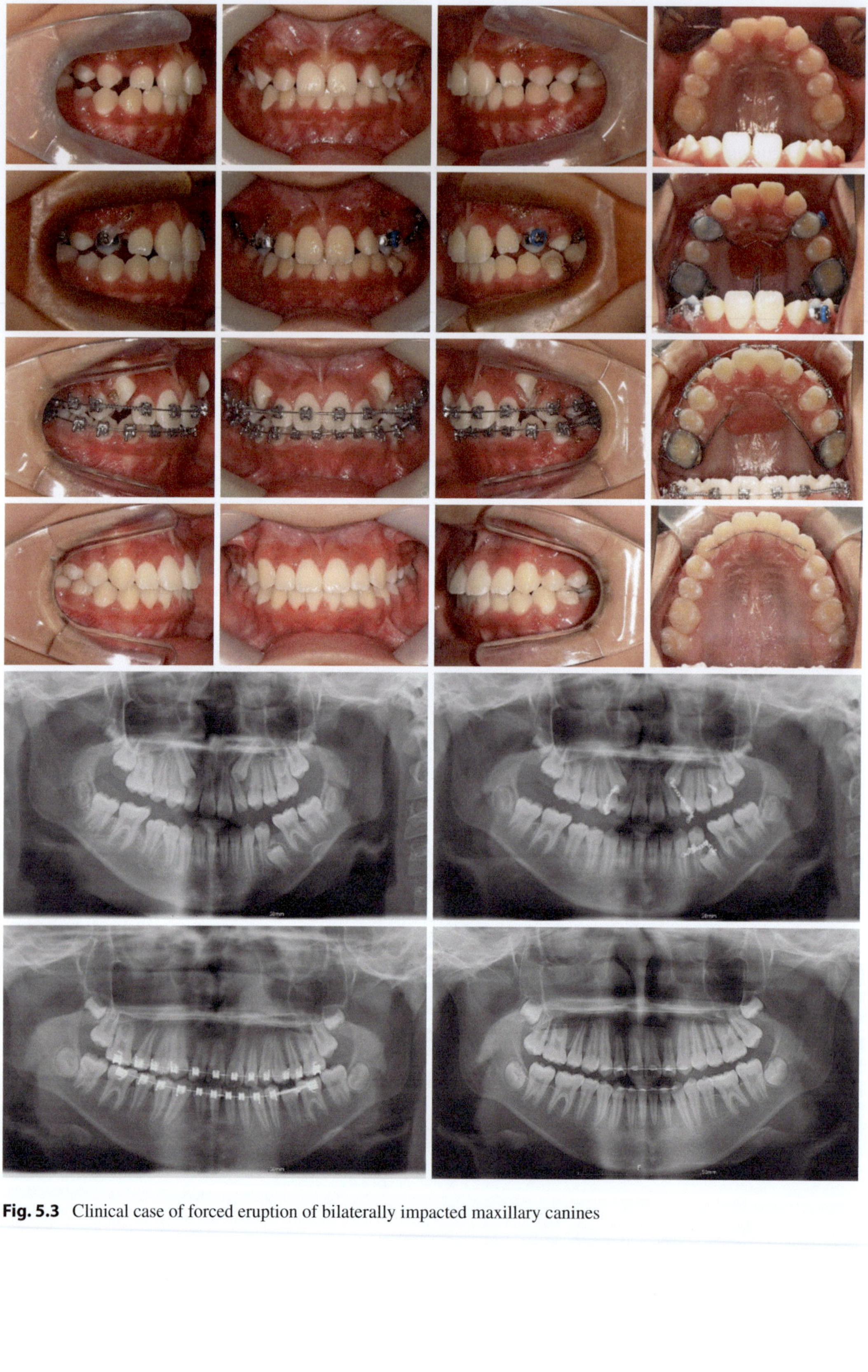

**Fig. 5.3** Clinical case of forced eruption of bilaterally impacted maxillary canines

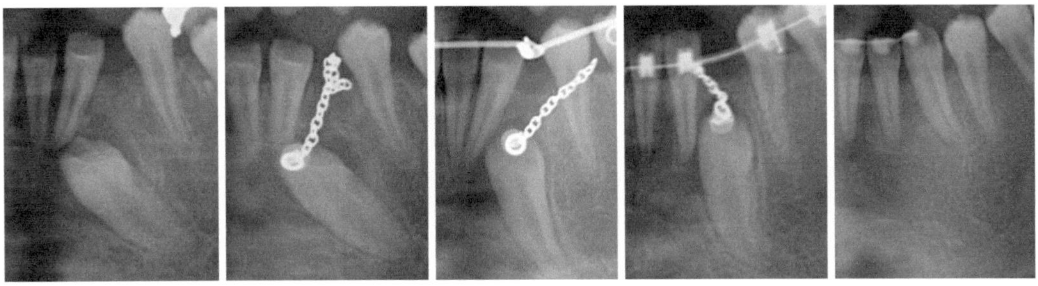

**Fig. 5.4** Forced eruption of impacted mandibular canine

3. Clinical case of forced eruption of impacted mandibular canine

   A 10-year and 2-month-old female patient presented with non-eruption of the left mandibular canine. Radiographic examination revealed impaction of left mandibular canine (Fig. 5.4). Under local anesthesia, and tooth #33 was treated with forced eruption instead of extraction. After initiating the forced eruption of #33, orthodontic treatment was conducted to create space for teeth #33. Two years post-surgery, satisfactory occlusion was achieved.
4. Impacted maxillary canine and premolars—multiple surgical exposure clinical case

   A 12-year and 7-month-old male patient presented with non-eruption of the left maxillary permanent teeth (Fig. 5.5). Radiographic examination revealed impaction of teeth #23, #24, and #25, with a dentigerous cyst observed above the crown of the impacted tooth #23. Cyst removal surgery was performed under general anesthesia, and tooth #23 was treated with forced eruption instead of extraction. After initiating the forced eruption of #23, orthodontic treatment was conducted to create space for teeth #24 and #25, followed by a stepwise forced eruption of these teeth. Five years post-surgery, there were no signs of cyst recurrence, and satisfactory occlusion was achieved.

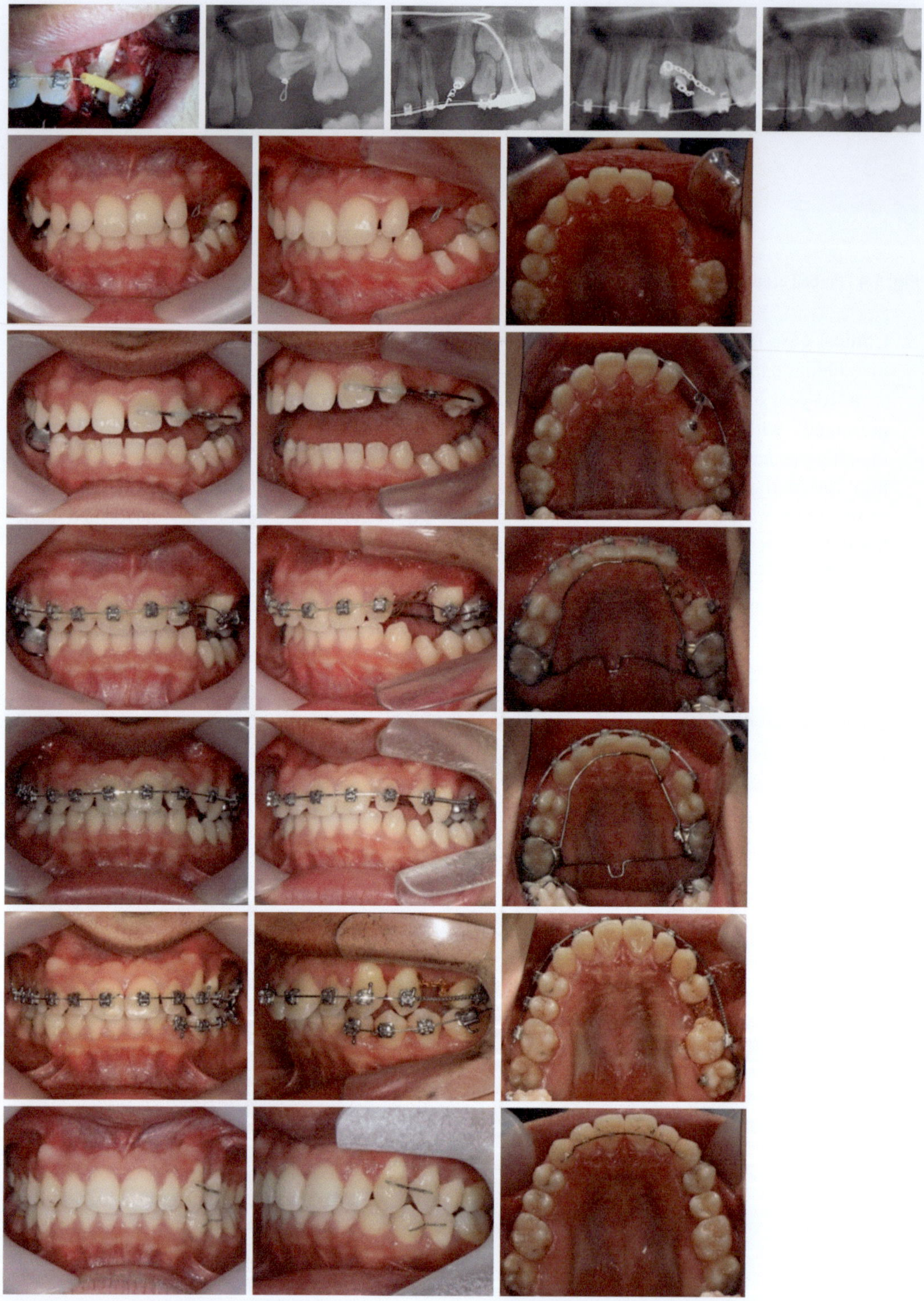

**Fig. 5.5** Impacted maxillary canine and premolars—multiple surgical exposure clinical case (by Courtesy of prof. Kim SH)

## 5.5 Conclusion

In this chapter, we have examined the prevalence, causes, and management of impacted canines. Detailed techniques for extraction, observation, and surgical exposure treatments have been described, each accompanied by each clinical case.

## References


1. Daskalogiannakis J. Multilingual glossary of orthodontic terms. Berlin: Quintessence Publishing Co; 2000.
2. Thilander B, Pena L, Infante C, Parada SS, de Mayorga C. Prevalence of malocclusion and orthodontic treatment need in children and adolescents in Bogota, Colombia. An epidemiological study related to different stages of dental development. Eur J Orthod. 2001;23(2):153–67. https://doi.org/10.1093/ejo/23.2.153.
3. Ericson S, Kurol J. Early treatment of palatally erupting maxillary canines by extraction of the primary canines. Eur J Orthod. 1983;10(4):283–95. https://doi.org/10.1093/ejo/10.4.283.
4. Jacoby H. The etiology of maxillary canine impactions. Am J Orthod. 1983;84(2):125–32. https://doi.org/10.1016/0002-9416(83)90176-8.
5. Kanavakis G, Curran KM, Wiseman KC, et al. Evaluation of crown-root angulation of lateral incisors adjacent to palatally impacted canines. Prog Orthod. 2015;16:4. https://doi.org/10.1186/s40510-015-0074-0.
6. Devi MSA, Padmanabhan S. Role of polymorphisms of MSX1 and PAX9 genes in palatal impaction of maxillary canines. J Orthod. 2019;46(1):14–9. https://doi.org/10.1177/1465312518820537.
7. Sathyanarayana HP, Nucci L, d'Apuzzo L, et al. Prevalence, etiology, clinical features and management associated with impacted and transmigrated mandibular canines: a systematic review. BMC Oral Health. 2023;23:975–91. https://doi.org/10.1186/s12903-023-03717-1.
8. Alqahtani H. Management of maxillary impacted canines: a prospective study of orthodontists' preferences. Saudi Pharm J. 2021;29(5):384–90. https://doi.org/10.1016/j.jsps.2021.03.010.

# 6 Surgical Extraction of Mandibular and Maxillary Third Molars

## Contents



## 6.1 Introduction

1. Overview of Third Molar Extraction

   Third molar extractions, commonly known as wisdom tooth removal, are among the most frequent surgical procedures in dental practice. These teeth, the last to emerge in the oral cavity, often present unique challenges due to their position and the time of their eruption. The extraction of third molars is significant due to its impact on oral health, including the prevention of overcrowding, infection, and other dental complications.

   The third molars are located at the farthest end of the dental arches, with two in the mandible (lower jaw) and two in the maxilla (upper jaw). These teeth are typically the last to erupt, usually during late adolescence or early adulthood. Due to their posterior position, they are more prone to problems such as impaction, where the tooth fails to emerge fully into its expected position, leading to a range of complications.
2. Indications for Surgical Extraction

   The decision to proceed with the surgical extraction of third molars is based on several criteria. These include the presence of impaction, recurrent infections like pericoronitis, cyst formation, potential damage to adjacent teeth, and orthodontic reasons [1].


S.-G. Kim et al., *Advanced Strategies for Tooth Extraction in Dentistry*,
https://doi.org/10.1007/978-981-97-6532-4_6

Additionally, prophylactic removal may be considered to prevent future complications, especially in cases where hygiene maintenance is challenging.

Surgical extraction differs from nonsurgical removal primarily in its approach and complexity. Nonsurgical extractions are performed when the tooth is fully erupted and visible in the mouth, requiring less invasive procedures. In contrast, surgical extraction is indicated when the tooth is impacted or partially erupted, involving incisions in the gum tissue and sometimes the removal of bone.

3. Anatomical Considerations

   Understanding the anatomy of the mandible and maxilla is crucial for safe and effective third molar extraction. This includes knowledge of the bone structure, the location of adjacent teeth, and the proximity to vital structures like nerves and blood vessels. The density and morphology of the jawbone can significantly influence the technique and approach of the extraction.

   Variability in root anatomy and nerve positioning, particularly the inferior alveolar nerve in the mandible, is a critical consideration. The roots of the third molars may be unusually shaped, multi-rooted, or positioned near nerves, increasing the complexity of the extraction and the risk of postoperative complications, such as nerve injury. Preoperative imaging and careful surgical planning are essential to minimize these risks.

## 6.2 Preoperative Assessment

### 6.2.1 Patient Evaluation

1. Medical History Considerations

   An exhaustive evaluation of the patient's medical history is a cornerstone of preoperative assessment for third molar extractions. This includes a detailed review of any systemic diseases, allergies, medications, and previous surgical experiences. Particular attention should be paid to conditions that may affect the surgical procedure or postoperative healing, such as diabetes, hypertension, bleeding disorders, and immune deficiencies. It is also vital to consider the patient's use of medications like anticoagulants or bisphosphonates, which can significantly impact bleeding risks and bone healing [2, 3]. An understanding of the patient's history aids in anticipating complications and planning an appropriate surgical approach.

2. Assessing Risk Factors

   Risk assessment is a critical aspect of preoperative evaluation, aiming to identify factors that may increase the complexity of the surgery or the likelihood of postoperative complications. This includes evaluating the anatomical positioning of the third molars, particularly the proximity to the inferior alveolar nerve in the mandible or the maxillary sinus in the upper jaw. Imaging studies, such as panoramic radiographs or cone beam computed tomography (CBCT), are instrumental in this assessment. Other risk factors include the patient's age, as older patients may experience more difficult recoveries, and the degree of impaction of the tooth, with deeper or more angular impactions presenting greater challenges. Here is a brief overview of the Pell and Gregory classification (Fig. 6.1) [4]:

   (a) Classification by Depth (Level)
      - Class A: The highest position of the impacted tooth is on the same level as the occlusal plane of the second molar.
      - Class B: The impacted tooth is between the occlusal plane of the second molar and the cervical line of the second molar.
      - Class C: The impacted tooth is below the cervical line of the second molar.

   (b) Classification by the Relationship to the Ramus of the Mandible
      - Class I: There is sufficient space between the ramus of the mandible and the second molar to accommodate the mesiodistal diameter of the crown of the impacted tooth.

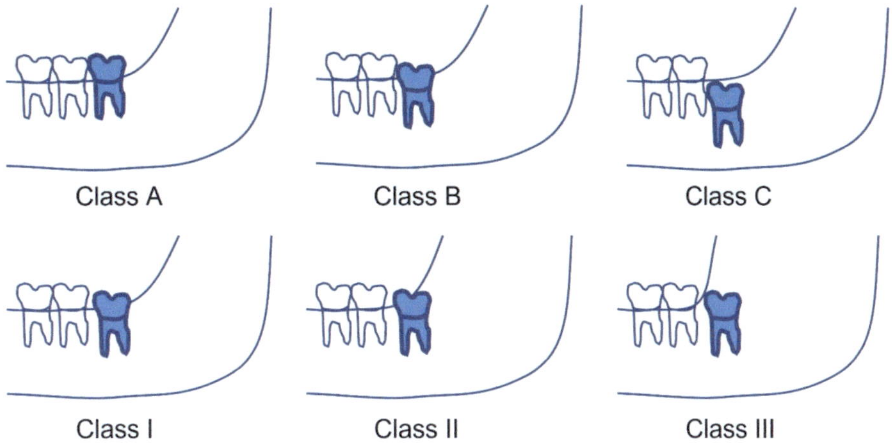


**Fig. 6.1** Pell and Gregory classification

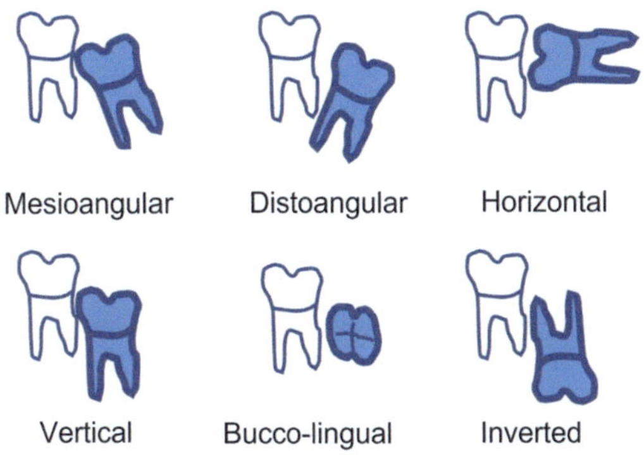


**Fig. 6.2** Winter's classification

- Class II: The space is less than the mesiodistal diameter of the crown of the impacted tooth.
- Class III: Most or all the tooth is within the ramus of the mandible.

The Winter's classification is based on tooth angulation (Fig. 6.2) [5]:

- Mesioangular: The most common type, where the tooth is angled toward the front of the mouth.
- Distoangular: The tooth is angled toward the back of the mouth.
- Horizontal: The tooth is lying on its side.
- Vertical: The tooth maintains a normal vertical position but is still impacted.
- Buccolingual: The tooth is angled perpendicularly or nearly perpendicularly to the dental arch, meaning it is oriented either toward the cheek (buccal) or toward the tongue (lingual).
- Inverted: The tooth is upside down.

Other risk factors can be anatomical positioning and patient's age.

- Anatomical positioning: This includes the proximity of the third molars to critical structures like the inferior alveolar nerve in the mandible and the maxillary sinus in the upper jaw. Advanced imaging techniques such as panoramic radiography or CBCT are invaluable in evaluating these relationships.
- Patient's age: Older patients may face more challenging recoveries, and the surgical approach may need to be adjusted accordingly [6].

The American Association of Oral and Maxillofacial Surgeons (AAOMS) recommends that wisdom teeth, also known as third molars, should ideally be extracted in the late teenage years to early twenties, generally before the roots are fully developed [6]. This typically occurs between the ages of 13 and 20. Extracting wisdom teeth at a younger age is often preferable because the long tooth roots have not fully developed, making the procedure simpler and recovery faster and more comfortable than removal at older ages when the tooth root and the jaw bone have fully matured. Most patients opt to have them out between the ages of 17 and 25 [6].

This recommendation is based on the understanding that younger patients often have a faster and more comfortable recovery process. As patients age, the roots of the wisdom teeth become fully developed and more firmly anchored in the jawbone, which can complicate the extraction process. Additionally, the jawbone in older patients is denser, which can make the surgery more challenging and increase the risk of complications. It is important to note that while these are general guidelines, the decision to remove wisdom teeth should be based on individual circumstances and a thorough evaluation by a dental professional. Each case should be assessed on its own merits, considering the patient's overall health, the condition of the teeth, and other relevant factors. By thoroughly assessing these risks, the dental surgeon can better prepare for the procedure and provide the patient with informed consent regarding potential complications and outcomes.

### 6.2.2 Diagnostic Imaging

1. Types of imaging and their roles
   (a) X-rays (Fig. 6.3a)

   X-rays, particularly panoramic radiographs (also known as orthopantomograms or OPGs), are the most used imaging technique in the assessment of third molars. They provide a broad view of the jaws, teeth, and surrounding structures. Panoramic X-rays are particularly useful for identifying the presence and position of impacted third molars, the relationship of the teeth to the mandibular canal and maxillary sinus, the extent of root development, and any pathology associated with the third molars [7, 8].

   (b) Cone Beam Computed Tomography (CBCT) (Fig. 6.3b–d)

   CBCT has become increasingly important in the evaluation of third molar impaction due to its ability to provide three-dimensional (3D) images. This technology offers detailed visualization of the spatial relationship between impacted teeth and critical structures like nerves and blood vessels. CBCT is especially valuable in complex cases where the proximity of the tooth to the inferior alveolar nerve or the morphology of the tooth roots may influence surgical planning [8].

   (c) Other Imaging Techniques

   While less common, other imaging modalities like traditional computed tomography (CT) scans or magnetic resonance imaging (MRI) can be used in specific scenarios [9]. CT scans can be helpful in complex maxillofacial trauma cases, while MRI might be used to assess soft tissue pathology or nerve involvement.

2. Interpreting Imaging for Surgical Planning

   The primary goal in interpreting imaging for third molar extraction is to understand the anatomical relationships between the impacted tooth and surrounding structures. Imaging helps in identifying the position of the tooth in relation to the mandibular canal, the maxillary sinus, and adjacent teeth [7–9]. This is crucial for minimizing the risk of nerve damage, particularly to the inferior alveolar nerve, and other complications during extraction.

Imaging plays a pivotal role in evaluating the type and depth of impaction, as classified by systems like Pell and Gregory [4] or Winter's [5]. This includes determining the angulation of the tooth, the depth of impaction relative to the occlusal plane, and the relationship to the mandibular ramus. Radiographs and CBCT can reveal pathologies such as cysts, tumors, or abnormal root development associated with third molars. Identifying these conditions preoperatively is essential for comprehensive treatment planning.

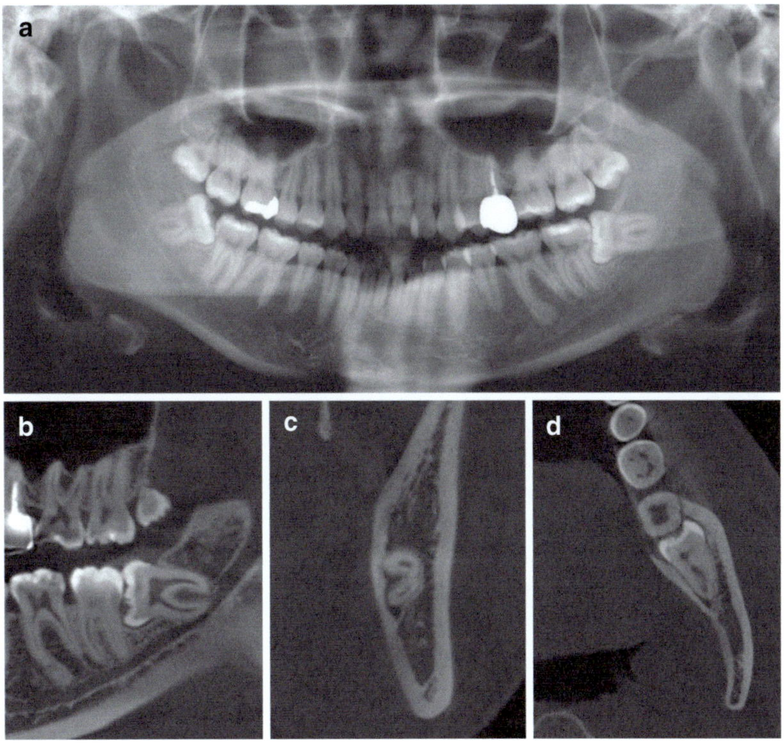


**Fig. 6.3** (**a**) Panoramic radiograph. (**b**) CBCT sagittal image, (**c**) CBCT coronal image, (**d**) CBCT axial image, all showing the left mandibular third molar

The insights gained from imaging guide the surgeon in planning the most appropriate surgical approach. This includes decisions about the type of incision, the need for bone removal, the possibility of tooth sectioning, and the approach to minimize trauma to surrounding tissues. Finally, diagnostic imaging aids in risk assessment and in informing the patient about the potential challenges and risks associated with the procedure. A thorough review of the imaging helps in obtaining informed consent by providing the patient with a clear understanding of their specific case.

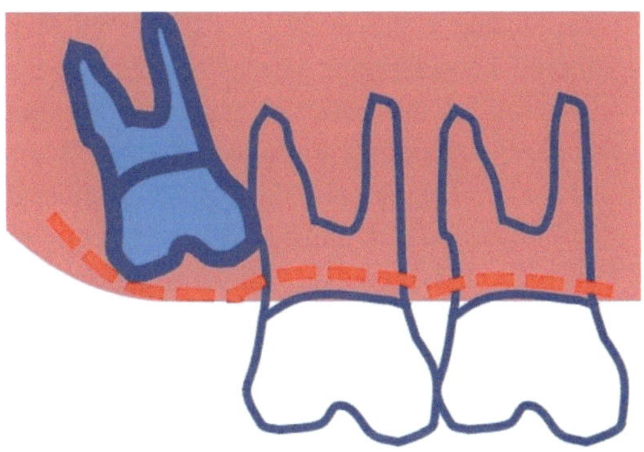

**Fig. 6.4** Envelope flap

## 6.3 Surgical Techniques

### 6.3.1 Maxillary Third Molars

1. Incision and flap design [10]
   (a) Standard approach (Fig. 6.4): A commonly used incision for maxillary third molar extraction is the envelope flap. This incision begins distally at the second molar and extends anteriorly along the alveolar ridge. It should be long enough to ensure good visibility and access to the third molar area.
   (b) Alternative approach (Fig. 6.5): For more complex cases, a three-cornered or triangular flap might be used. This involves an additional vertical releasing incision, which can provide better exposure, especially in cases of impacted molars.

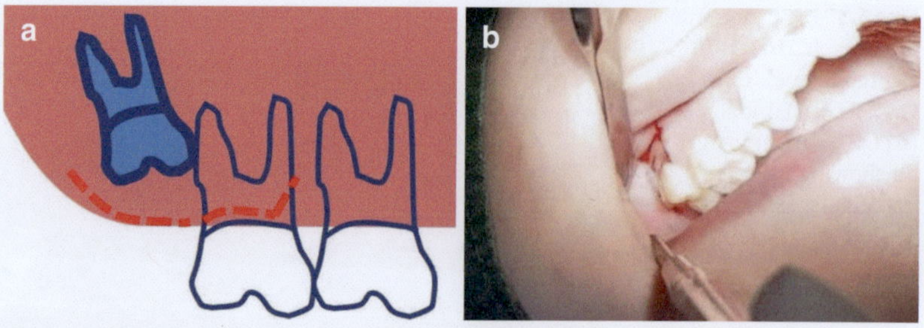


**Fig. 6.5** (**a**) Triangular flap, (**b**) incision

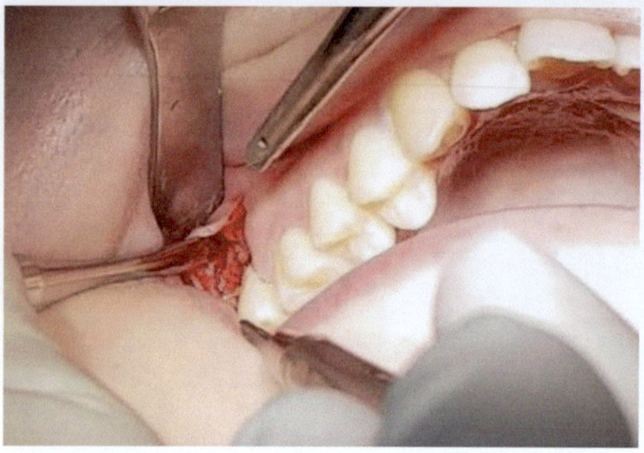

**Fig. 6.6** Flap elevation

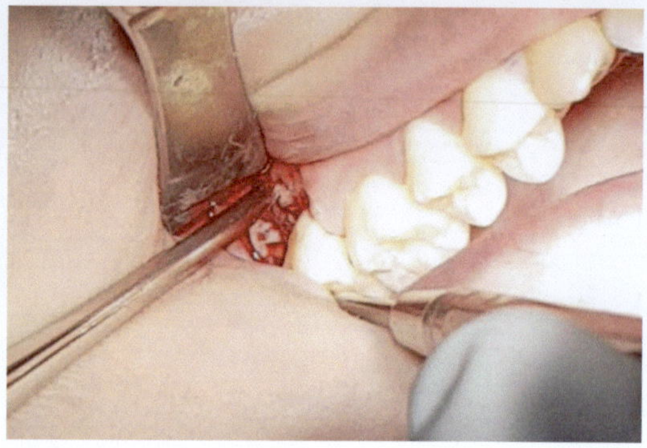

**Fig. 6.7** Extraction using straight elevator

2. Flap elevation (Fig. 6.6): Carefully elevate the flap using a periosteal elevator. This step should be performed gently to preserve the integrity of the periosteum and to prevent unnecessary trauma to the overlying soft tissue. The elevation should expose the buccal bone overlying the third molar sufficiently to allow for its removal and the subsequent extraction of the tooth.
3. Bone removal: The bone covering the impacted maxillary third molar is removed using a surgical handpiece with bur or bone chisel. A portion of the crown is exposed by removing the thinnest part of the bone covering the crown of the impacted tooth, and the removal of bone continues until the maximum contour of the tooth crown is completely exposed.
4. Extraction using elevator (Fig. 6.7): After exposing the impacted tooth, create a space on the bucco-mesial side of the impacted tooth, between the crown and the surrounding bone, for the insertion of an elevator. Insert the elevator into the created space and extract the impacted tooth from its position to distally and downward. During this process, exercise caution by palpating the maxillary second molar with a finger to ensure it does not become dislodged during the extraction of the impacted tooth.
5. Debridement: After the extraction, thoroughly debride the socket to remove any loose bone fragments, which helps in reducing postoperative complications.
6. Suturing (Fig. 6.8): After the extraction, the flap must be repositioned and secured with sutures. The choice of suture material and technique depends on the clinician's preference and the specific requirements of the case. Proper suturing is crucial to ensure primary closure of the wound, reduce the risk of infection, and promote healing.

### 6.3.2 Specific Challenges and Solutions in Maxillary Third Molars

1. Limited Access and Visibility
   (a) Challenge: The maxillary third molars are located at the back of the mouth, making them difficult to access and visualize during extraction.

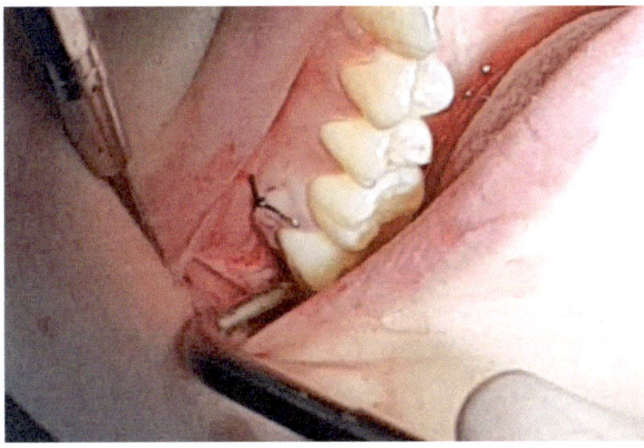

**Fig. 6.8** Suturing

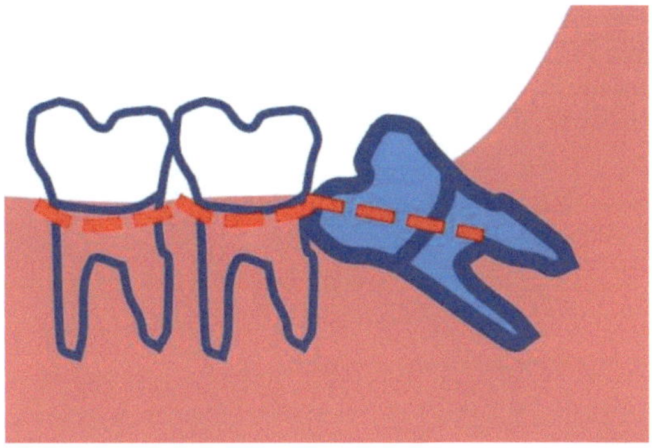

**Fig. 6.9** Envelope flap

   (b) Solution: Use mouth props and cheek retractors to improve visibility and access. Also, selecting the appropriate flap design, as discussed earlier, can significantly enhance access to the surgical area.
2. Proximity to the Maxillary Sinus
   (a) Challenge: The roots of the maxillary third molars can be close to or protrude into the maxillary sinus, posing a risk of sinus perforation.
   (b) Solution: Careful preoperative evaluation, including radiographic analysis, is crucial. During extraction, gentle techniques should be used to avoid excessive force that could lead to sinus membrane perforation.
3. Anatomical Variations
   (a) Challenge: Variations in root anatomy, such as curved or multiple roots, can complicate extractions.
   (b) Solution: Detailed radiographic assessment is essential to understand root morphology. Modify extraction techniques based on the anatomical presentation of each case.
4. Risk of Damage to Adjacent Teeth
   (a) Challenge: There is a risk of damaging the adjacent second molar, particularly its crown or roots.
   (b) Solution: Ensure that the instruments used for elevation and extraction are appropriately positioned and manipulated. The use of specialized instruments, like a straight elevator, can minimize this risk.

### 6.3.3 Mandibular Third Molars

1. Incision and flap design [10]
   (a) Standard approach (Fig. 6.9): A commonly used incision for mandibular third molars is the envelope or Ward's incision. This incision typically starts at the distal aspect of the second molar and extends posteriorly and slightly distally, following the external oblique ridge.
   (b) Alternative approach (Fig. 6.10): For impacted teeth or when greater access is needed, a modified Ward's incision with a distal releasing incision can be used. This additional incision extends vertically down the ramus of the mandible, providing broader access.
2. Flap elevation (Fig. 6.11): Gently elevate the mucoperiosteal flap using a periosteal elevator, being careful to maintain the integrity of the periosteum for effective healing post-extraction. The elevation should expose the external oblique ridge and provide sufficient visibility and access to the impacted tooth.
3. Bone removal (Fig. 6.12): Using a surgical handpiece and bur, remove the bone overlying the tooth, particularly on the buccal side. The goal is to expose enough of the crown and root to facilitate extraction.

**Fig. 6.10** Modified Ward's incision. (**a**) schematic illustration, (**b**) intraoral application

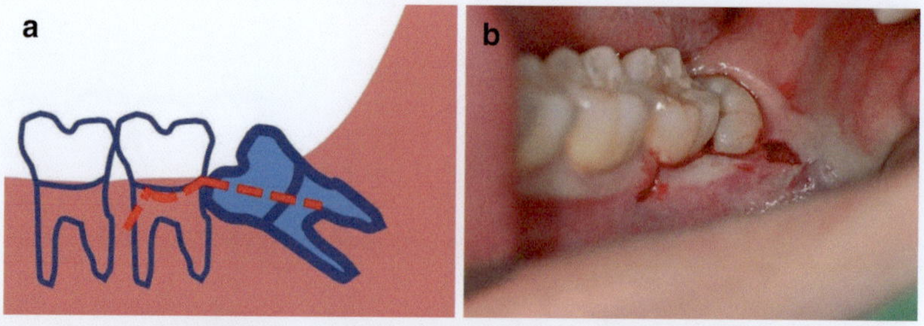


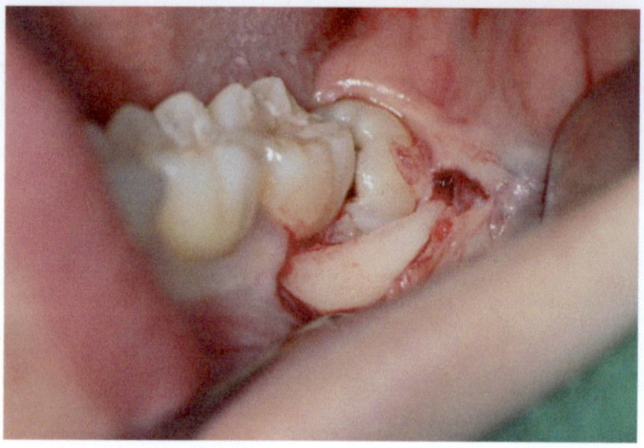

**Fig. 6.11** Flap elevation

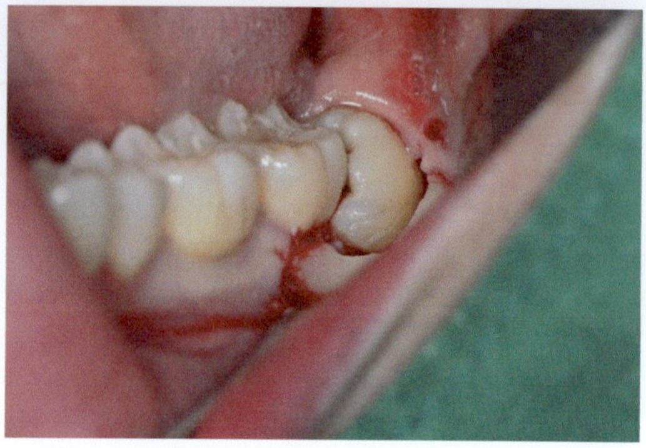

**Fig. 6.12** Buccal bone removal

4. Tooth Sectioning
   (a) When to section: Tooth sectioning is often necessary when the tooth is impacted, or its roots are divergent, hooked, or near the inferior alveolar nerve.
   (b) Sectioning Technique
      - Crown sectioning: Make an initial cut through the crown of the tooth, dividing it into two or more sections. This facilitates the removal of each section separately (Fig. 6.13a).
      - Root sectioning: In cases with complex root anatomy, section the roots after crown removal. This allows each root to be removed individually, reducing the risk of damage to the mandibular canal (Fig. 6.13b).
5. Extraction using elevator: Once sectioned, use elevators to gently luxate and remove each piece. Be cautious to apply controlled force to avoid fracturing the roots or damaging adjacent structures.
6. Debridement and suturing (Fig. 6.14).

### 6.3.4 Managing Impactions and Difficult Extractions in Mandibular Third Molars

Deeply impacted and ankylosed mandibular third molars require specialized surgical techniques due to their complexity. Here is a detailed approach to these specific cases.

1. Deeply Impacted Teeth
   (a) Preoperative Assessment
      - Radiographic analysis: Utilize detailed imaging like CBCT scans to assess the depth of impaction, root anatomy, and proximity to the inferior alveolar nerve.
      - Surgical planning: Plan the surgery considering the likelihood of needing extensive bone removal and potential nerve involvement.
   (b) Surgical Technique
      - Access and bone removal: Create a larger flap for better access. Remove

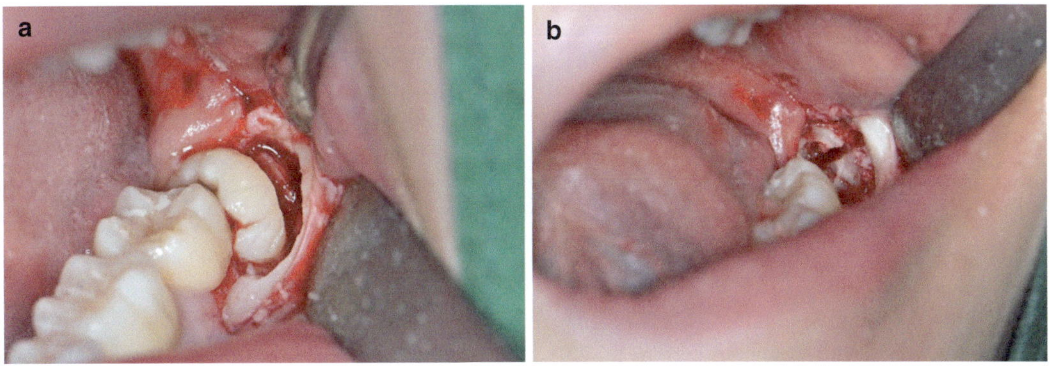

Fig. 6.13 Tooth sectioning. (a) Crown sectioning, (b) root sectioning

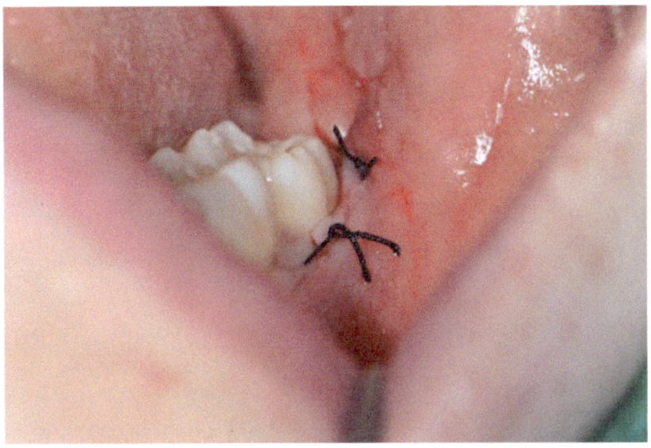

Fig. 6.14 Suturing

bone carefully around the tooth, ensuring not to damage the inferior alveolar nerve.
  - Sectioning: Section the tooth to facilitate removal in parts. In cases close to the nerve, consider coronectomy (removing the crown while leaving the roots in situ) to minimize the risk of nerve damage.

(c) Handling Nerve Exposure: If the nerve is exposed or involved, handle it gently. In some cases, it might be prudent to leave a small part of the root to avoid nerve injury.

2. Ankylosed Teeth
   (a) Identification: Ankylosed teeth are characterized by the fusion of the tooth to the surrounding bone, making them challenging to extract.
   (b) Surgical Approach
   - Incision and flap design: A broad flap may be necessary to provide sufficient visibility and access.
   - Bone removal: Carefully remove bone around the tooth. Due to the fusion, more bone removal than usual may be required.
   - Sectioning and elevation: Section the tooth if possible. Use surgical burs to cut through the ankylosis areas. Elevation can be challenging; apply steady and controlled forces to avoid fracturing the jaw.

   (c) Socket Management: After removal, thoroughly clean the socket to remove any remaining ankylosed bone fragments. Consider bone grafting if there is significant bone loss.

## 6.4 Postoperative Care

1. Postoperative Care Guidelines

   The postoperative phase is critical in ensuring a smooth recovery and minimizing complications following third molar surgery. Effective postoperative care involves several key guidelines.

   (a) Pain management: Patients are often prescribed pain relievers, such as NSAIDs or

acetaminophen, to manage discomfort. In cases of more severe pain, a short course of stronger analgesics may be prescribed.
   (b) Swelling and bruising control: Swelling is common after third molar extraction. Patients are advised to use ice packs on the cheek in the first 24 h to reduce swelling. Bruising may also occur, which typically resolves on its own.
   (c) Oral hygiene: Maintaining oral hygiene is crucial for preventing infection. Patients should be instructed on gentle cleaning techniques around the surgical site, avoiding vigorous rinsing or spitting in the initial days.
   (d) Diet: A soft or liquid diet is recommended initially, gradually returning to normal as comfort allows. Hot and spicy foods should be avoided as they can irritate the wound site.
   (e) Activity restrictions: Patients should avoid strenuous activities for a few days post-surgery to reduce the risk of bleeding and enhance healing.
   (f) Wound care: If sutures are placed, instructions on their care or removal (if not self-dissolving) should be provided.
   (g) Signs of complications: Patients should be educated about signs of possible complications, such as excessive bleeding, persistent pain, swelling, fever, or signs of infection, and instructed to contact the dental office if these occur.
2. Scheduling Follow-up Visits and What to Monitor
   (a) Initial follow-up: The first follow-up is usually scheduled within a week post-surgery to monitor the healing process, assess pain management, and remove sutures if necessary.
   (b) Monitoring healing: During follow-up visits, the surgical site is examined for signs of proper healing, infection, or other complications.
   (c) Pain and swelling evaluation: Persistent pain or swelling beyond the expected time frame should be evaluated to rule out complications like dry socket or infection.
   (d) Oral hygiene and diet progress: The dentist or oral surgeon assesses the patient's ability to maintain oral hygiene and transition back to a normal diet, providing additional guidance as needed.
   (e) Long-term follow-up: In some cases, especially if there were complications or the patient has specific health concerns, additional follow-up appointments may be scheduled.

These postoperative care guidelines and follow-up schedules are designed to ensure optimal recovery, identify, and address any complications early, and provide the patient with support and information throughout the healing process. Tailoring these guidelines to individual patient needs and circumstances is vital for successful postoperative management.

## 6.5 Conclusion

This chapter comprehensively addressed the multifaceted aspects of surgical extraction of mandibular and maxillary third molars. Key points included the intricate preoperative assessments, the diverse techniques and challenges of surgical extractions, and the pivotal role of anesthesia and pain control. Special emphasis was placed on intraoperative management, highlighting hemostasis, infection control, and patient monitoring. The chapter also covered postoperative care and the importance of follow-up visits.

Looking ahead, the chapter anticipates ongoing advancements in techniques and technologies in third molar extraction. These developments are expected to refine best practices and improve patient outcomes. The evolving landscape of dental surgery demands continuous learning and adaptation to emerging trends and innovations. This conclusion encapsulates the essence of the chapter, underlining the critical importance of skill, knowledge, and adaptability in the field of dental surgery, particularly in the complex task of third molar extractions.

## References

1. Kandasamy S, Rinchuse DJ, Rinchuse DJ. The wisdom behind third molar extractions. Aust Dent J. 2009;54(4):284–92. https://doi.org/10.1111/j.1834-7819.2009.01152.x.
2. Abdullah WA, Khalil H. Dental extraction in patients on warfarin treatment. Clin Cosmet Investig Dent. 2014;6:65–9. https://doi.org/10.2147/CCIDE.S68641.
3. Ruggiero SL, Dodson TB, Aghaloo T, Carlson ER, Ward BB, Kademani D. American Association of Oral and Maxillofacial Surgeons' position paper on medication-related osteonecrosis of the Jaws-2022 update. J Oral Maxillofac Surg. 2022;80(5):920–43. https://doi.org/10.1016/j.joms.2022.02.008.
4. Pell GJ, Gregory BT. Impacted mandibular third molars: classification and modified techniques for removal. Dent Digest. 1933;39:330–8.
5. Winter GB. Impacted mandibular third molars. St Louis: American Medical Book Co.; 1926.
6. Pogrel MA, Dodson TB, Swift JQ, et al. White paper on third molar data. 2007 [cited 2023 Dec 13]. https://www.aaoms.org/docs/govt_affairs/advocacy_white_papers/white_paper_third_molar_data.pdf
7. Seo MH, Sodnom-Ish B, Eo MY, Myoung H, Kim SM. Radiographic evaluation before surgical extraction of impacted third molar to reduce the maxillary sinus related complication. J Korean Assoc Oral Maxillofac Surg. 2023;49(4):192–7. https://doi.org/10.5125/jkaoms.2023.49.4.192.
8. Patel PS, Shah JS, Dudhia BB, Butala PB, Jani YV, Macwan RS. Comparison of panoramic radiograph and cone beam computed tomography findings for impacted mandibular third molar root and inferior alveolar nerve canal relation. Indian J Dent Res. 2020;31(1):91–102. https://doi.org/10.4103/ijdr.IJDR_540_18.
9. Ferretti F, Malventi M, Malasoma R. Dental magnetic resonance imaging: study of impacted mandibular third molars. Dentomaxillofac Radiol. 2009;38(6):387–92. https://doi.org/10.1259/dmfr/29929241.
10. Sifuentes-Cervantes JS, Carrillo-Morales F, Castro-Nunez J, Cunningham LL, Van Sickels JE. Third molar surgery: past, present, and the future. Oral Surg Oral Med Oral Pathol Oral Radiol. 2021;132(5):523–31. https://doi.org/10.1016/j.oooo.2021.03.004.

# Management of Complications in Tooth Extraction

7

## Contents



## 7.1 Introduction

Tooth extraction, a common dental procedure, involves the removal of a tooth from its socket in the bone. It is typically performed when a tooth is damaged beyond repair due to decay, periodontal disease, or trauma. Tooth extraction can be categorized into two main types: simple extractions and surgical extractions. Simple extractions are usually performed on teeth that are visible in the mouth. These procedures are typically straightforward; the dentist uses an instrument called an elevator to loosen the tooth and forceps to remove it. On the other hand, surgical extractions involve





S.-G. Kim et al., *Advanced Strategies for Tooth Extraction in Dentistry*,
https://doi.org/10.1007/978-981-97-6532-4_7

removing teeth that are not easily accessible. This could be because they have not erupted fully or they have broken under the gum line. In these cases, the dentist may need to cut and pull back the gums, removing bone tissue or breaking the tooth into smaller pieces to extract it.

The process of tooth extraction begins with a thorough evaluation, including a review of the patient's medical history and appropriate imaging studies, like X-rays. Local anesthesia is commonly administered to numb the area around the tooth to minimize discomfort. Post-procedure, patients are provided with guidelines to follow during the healing process, which is crucial for preventing complications. While tooth extraction is generally safe, it can lead to complications, which, though rare, can be significant. The management of these complications is paramount in dental practice for several reasons. Firstly, immediate management of complications like bleeding, swelling, and infection is crucial for patient comfort and health. Uncontrolled bleeding can lead to anemia or other serious conditions, and infections, if left untreated, can spread to other parts of the body. Nerve damage, another possible complication, can result in prolonged numbness or pain.

Additionally, effective complication management is vital for maintaining patient trust and the professional reputation of the dental practice. Complications that are not promptly or adequately addressed can lead to patient dissatisfaction, negative reviews, and even legal issues. Moreover, understanding and managing these complications underscores the importance of proper pre-extraction evaluation and planning. It highlights the need for dentists to be vigilant and proactive in identifying potential risks and taking steps to mitigate them. This includes a comprehensive understanding of the patient's medical history, the structure of the affected tooth, and the surrounding bone and gum tissue.

In summary, the management of complications in tooth extraction is not only about addressing problems after they arise but also about preventing them wherever possible. This proactive approach ensures patient safety, promotes faster healing, and upholds the standards of dental care.

## 7.2 Prevalence and Risk Factors for Complications

### 7.2.1 Statistics on Complications Following Tooth Extractions

The incidence of complications following tooth extractions varies, but understanding these statistics is crucial for dentists to anticipate, prevent, and manage these complications effectively. A comprehensive study revealed that the overall complication rate in tooth extractions was approximately 4.6% [1]. Most of these complications were of an inflammatory nature, with alveolitis emerging as the most common issue [1, 2]. Moreover, the operative complication rate, which includes issues encountered during the extraction procedure itself, stood at 1.2%, with bleeding being the most frequent operative complication [1]. Significantly, factors such as the patient's age and their medical history positively correlated with an increased risk of complications [1].

When focusing on wisdom tooth extractions, one of the predominant complications identified is infection [2]. This can present in various forms, including swelling, pain, abscess formation, fever, or the development of a dry socket, a painful condition where a blood clot fails to form or is dislodged from the extraction site [2]. In a broader context, the range of complications post-tooth extraction can include alveolitis, hemorrhage, wound dehiscence, and even fracture of the bone cortices [3]. Although tooth extraction is a routine dental procedure, the incidence of complications reported in studies varies significantly, ranging from 1% to a high of 30.9% [3].

A specific study examining 598 tooth extractions, encompassing both routine and surgical procedures, found that postoperative complications occurred in 12.4% of cases [4]. The most common complications in this cohort were dry socket and postoperative pain, highlighting the need for careful management and follow-up [4]. Additionally, in scenarios where tooth extractions were performed under general anesthesia, the complication rates differed based on the location of the tooth. The complication rate for lower third molars was 8.2%, compared to only 1.5% for upper third molars [5]. This study also pointed out that complications were more frequent when the procedure was performed by a less experienced operator, the patient was older, or the tooth was deeply embedded, underscoring the importance of experience and patient evaluation in minimizing complications [5]. While tooth extractions are generally safe, the range of possible complications and their varying incidence rates underscore the importance of thorough preoperative assessment, skilled surgical technique, and diligent postoperative care to mitigate these risks.

### 7.2.2 Identifying High-Risk Patients and Situations

Recognizing patients and situations that present a higher risk of complications during tooth extractions is a critical aspect of dental care.

1. Preoperative Risks

   Medical history and current medications are crucial to evaluate. Bisphosphonates, commonly used for osteoporosis or cancer treatment, can hinder the healing process [6]. A history of radiation therapy in the head and neck increases the risk of osteoradionecrosis, characterized by bone death due to damaged blood vessels [7]. Difficulty in achieving effective anesthesia, coupled with poor patient cooperation, can pose significant challenges. These factors may necessitate specialized care or modifications in treatment planning [8]. Limited mouth opening (trismus), microstomia, or crowded teeth may require a more complex surgical approach, thereby increasing the risk of complications [8].
2. Intraoperative Risks

   A thorough assessment of the tooth and root structure, both clinically and through X-rays, helps predict potential issues. Complex root structures or teeth embedded in dense bone may complicate the extraction process [9]. Fracturing the tooth, socket, or jawbone is a concern, especially in osteoporotic patients or in cases where the tooth has extensive decay or restorations [10]. The risk of nerve damage, leading to numbness or tingling sensations, is particularly high in lower wisdom tooth extractions or where significant bone removal near nerve locations is required [11].
3. Postoperative Risks

   Excessive bleeding is more likely in patients on anticoagulants or those with bleeding disorders [12]. Infection risks are heightened in immunocompromised individuals, including those with conditions like diabetes or HIV [13]. Dry socket, a condition where the blood clot at the extraction site is dislodged, and other healing complications can arise, influenced by factors such as the extraction type and postoperative care. Post-extraction, teeth may shift, leading to misalignment and bite changes. This is particularly concerning if back teeth are removed, potentially necessitating further dental interventions or orthodontic corrections. A detailed understanding of a patient's medical background, dental anatomy, and specific extraction-related factors is vital. This knowledge assists in customizing the approach to each extraction, minimizing risks, and ensuring safer dental procedures.

## 7.3 Common Complications

### 7.3.1 Bleeding

Bleeding is a common complication following tooth extraction, and managing it effectively is crucial for patient safety and comfort (Fig. 7.1). This section explores the causes, preventive measures, and management strategies for bleeding post-tooth extraction, guided by recent scientific literature.

1. Causes

   Bleeding after tooth extraction can occur due to various reasons. In some cases, it is related to the patient's inherent conditions, such as coagulation disorders like hemophilia, von Willebrand's disease, or systemic conditions like afibrinogenemia [14]. Certain medications, particularly anticoagulants, significantly increase the risk of bleeding [15]. For instance, patients on anticoagulant therapy with vitamin K antagonists (VKAs) or non-vitamin K antagonists present different levels of bleeding risk during dental surgeries (Table 7.1).

2. Prevention

   Preventive measures are vital in minimizing the risk of bleeding. A thorough preoperative assessment, including a detailed medical history and current medication review, is essential. For patients with known coagulation disorders, pretreatment with specific agents such as fibrinogen concentrate in afibrinogenemia may be necessary [16]. Additionally, dental professionals should be aware of conditions like mild hemophilia, which may remain asymptomatic and undiagnosed until adulthood, as standard coagulation tests might not always reveal these conditions [17].

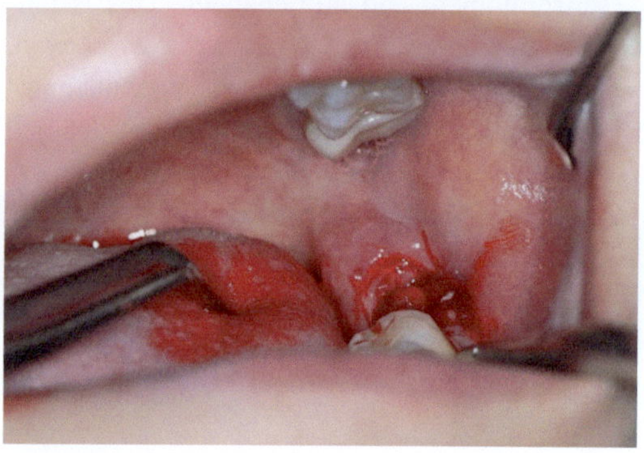

**Fig. 7.1** Bleeding after extraction. Patient received gelatin sponge application for bleeding control

3. Management Strategies

   Effective management of post-extraction bleeding involves a combination of local and systemic measures. For patients on anticoagulant therapy, using autologous platelet concentrates has been shown to be an effective hemostatic agent [12]. This approach balances the need to control bleeding with the risk of thromboembolic events due to altering anticoagulant therapy. The application of hemostatic agents after tooth extractions is another critical strategy (Fig. 7.2). A systematic review and meta-analysis by Mahardawi B et al. [18] highlight various agents' roles in controlling post-extraction bleeding. The study provides a comprehensive overview of their effectiveness, aiding in informed decision-making for bleeding management. In specific cases, such as hemophilia or other bleeding disorders, collaboration with hematologists for specialized care, including factor replacement therapy, is necessary [19]. Understanding the unique challenges of these conditions ensures tailored management for each patient.

**Table 7.1** Anticoagulant drugs and their potential bleeding risk after tooth extraction

| Anticoagulant drug | Potential bleeding risk (post-extraction) | Notes |
|---|---|---|
| Warfarin | Comparable to DOACs | Requires the same level of caution as DOACs for tooth extractions |
| Direct oral anticoagulants (DOACs) | Comparable to warfarin | Includes drugs like apixaban, dabigatran, edoxaban, rivaroxaban |
| Vitamin K inhibitors | Higher compared to non-AT patients | Significantly increased risk of postoperative bleeding |
| Apixaban | Lower than rivaroxaban, higher than edoxaban and dabigatran | Moderate risk |
| Dabigatran | Lowest (no incidents reported in the study) | Safest among the listed drugs in terms of bleeding risk |
| Edoxaban | Lower than rivaroxaban and Apixaban | Relatively low risk |
| Rivaroxaban | Highest among the studied anticoagulants | Significantly higher risk of postoperative bleeding |

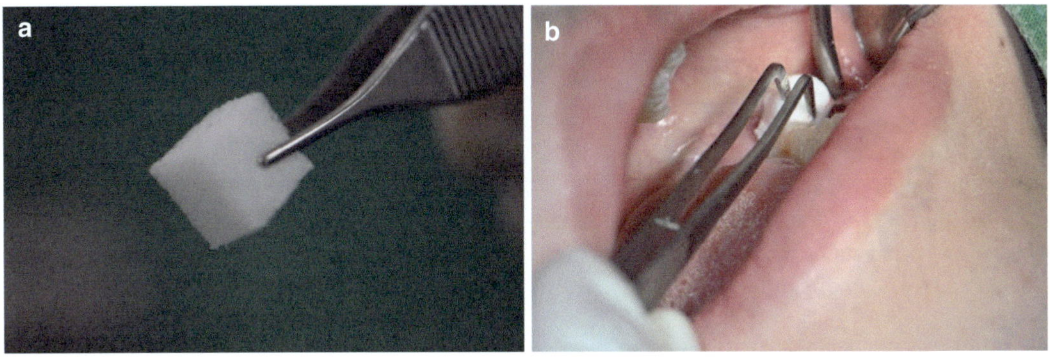

**Fig. 7.2** The application of hemostat. (**a**) Gelatin sponge, (**b**) the application of gelatin sponge

Managing bleeding after tooth extraction requires an understanding of the underlying causes, risk factors, and effective utilization of preventive and therapeutic measures. The integration of recent scientific findings into clinical practice enhances the safety and efficacy of dental procedures, particularly in high-risk patients. Regular updates to these practices, in line with evolving research, are essential for optimal patient care.

### 7.3.2 Swelling

Swelling is a common complication following the extraction of impacted teeth, often accompanied by pain and edema [20]. This phenomenon is a natural response to the tissue trauma incurred during the surgical procedure (Fig. 7.3). As one of the most frequent operations performed by oral and maxillofacial surgeons, managing these postoperative symptoms is crucial for patient comfort and recovery [20]. Manual lymph drainage (MLD) has been explored as a method to reduce postoperative facial swelling and discomfort [21]. A study involving ten patients undergoing bilateral wisdom tooth removal found MLD to be effective in mitigating swelling, highlighting its potential as a therapeutic approach in dental surgery [21].

Another promising treatment is low-level laser therapy (LLLT). Research has shown that LLLT, particularly when applied to impacted molars and associated postoperative pain, can be a beneficial intervention [22]. This therapy aids in the prevention and control of postoperative complications, including trismus, a common issue following tooth extraction [22]. The use of antibiotics has also been investigated to prevent complications such as dry socket, a painful condition following tooth extraction [23]. Studies suggest that antibiotics can reduce the incidence of dry socket by 34%, providing a significant preventive measure against this postoperative complication [23].

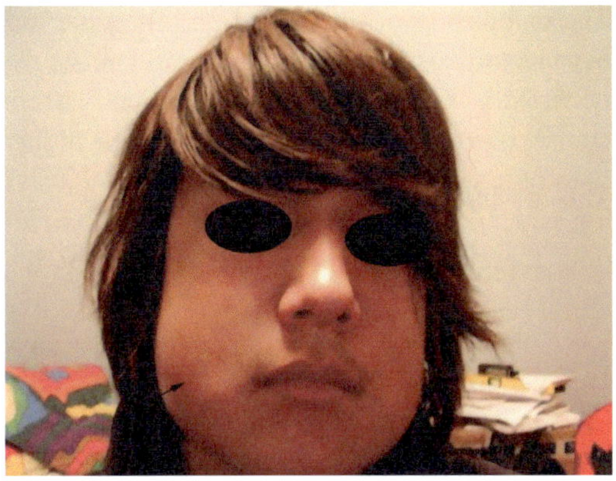

**Fig. 7.3** Severe facial swelling after right mandibular third molar extraction (arrow)

Other studies have focused on different approaches, like the use of hyaluronic acid sprays [24] and cold treatments [25]. Hyaluronic acid sprays have been shown to effectively reduce swelling, pain, and trismus in patients after impacted mandibular third molar extraction [24]. Similarly, the application of cold treatment post-surgery has been reported to have beneficial effects on swelling, edema, and pain, further aiding in reducing bleeding and hematomas [25].

The management of swelling after tooth extraction requires a multifaceted approach. Techniques such as MLD, LLLT, antibiotic prophylaxis, hyaluronic acid sprays, and cold treatment offer varied but effective means of reducing postoperative complications and enhancing patient recovery.

**Table 7.2** Risk factors for delayed-onset infection (DOI) after wisdom tooth extraction

| Risk factor | Description |
| --- | --- |
| Winter classification | The position of the wisdom tooth, with Class III (deeper impaction) associated with higher DOI risk |
| Hypertension | Patients with hypertension showing a higher incidence of DOI |
| Hemostatic agent | Usage of oxidized cellulose as a hemostatic agent linked to an increased risk of DOI, possibly due to bacterial attachment to the agent |

### 7.3.3 Infection

The complexity of the extraction procedure has been identified as a primary factor influencing the occurrence of postoperative infections. More complex extractions are associated with higher rates of infection. In a retrospective study involving patients who underwent third molar extraction, the complexity of the extraction was the only variable that significantly affected the occurrence of postoperative infection, as indicated by a binary logistic regression (OR = 2.03, $p = 0.004$) [2]. Additionally, another study aimed to identify the risk factors for postoperative infections, particularly after third molar extraction surgery, and to distinguish between early- and delayed-onset infections [26].

Recognizing the signs of postoperative infection is crucial for timely intervention. Infections can manifest in various forms, ranging from localized swelling and pain to more severe symptoms such as fever and pus discharge. Timely diagnosis and appropriate antibiotic therapy are key in managing these infections. A study among veterans detailed the antibiotic prescribing patterns and the incidence of and risk factors for post-extraction oral infection, providing insights into effective management strategies [27].

The use of antibiotics to prevent postoperative complications, including infections, has been extensively debated. Some studies suggest that antibiotics may reduce the risk of complications like dry socket, which, while not directly an infection, can be a gateway for bacterial invasion if not properly managed [23]. Additionally, maintaining strict aseptic techniques during and after the extraction procedure plays a crucial role in preventing infection. A specific concern in dental extractions is delayed-onset infection (DOI), which can occur approximately 1–4 weeks post-extraction [13]. A study that analyzed cases of mandibular wisdom tooth extractions identified several risk factors for DOI (Table 7.2), highlighting the need for careful postoperative monitoring and follow-up [13].

In summary, the management of post-extraction infections encompasses a broad spectrum of practices, from assessing risk factors and signs to implementing effective prevention and treatment strategies. The complexity of the extraction, adherence to aseptic techniques, and judicious use of antibiotics are all pivotal in minimizing the risk of infection and ensuring patient safety and comfort.

### 7.3.4 Nerve Damage

Nerve injury in dentistry, particularly following tooth extraction, is a significant concern due to its potential to cause lasting discomfort and impairment. Various dental procedures, including extraction, have been identified as potential causes of injury to the oral branches of the trigeminal nerve. These injuries can result from local anesthetic injections, root canal therapy, implant insertion, bone grafting, and dentoalveolar surgery, all of which necessitate careful procedural planning and execution to minimize risk [28].

Symptoms of nerve damage can range from numbness and tingling to severe pain and hypersensitivity. Mental nerve neuropathy, also known as numb chin syndrome, is an uncommon but notable condition following dental extraction, characterized by altered sensation or pain in the chin and lower lip area. It is essential for such neuropathies to be diagnosed accurately to avoid unnecessary treatments and further complications [29, 30]. Prevention of nerve injury hinges on accurate diagnosis, meticulous surgical technique, and patient education. For instance, the early diagnosis of orthodontic-related nerve injuries can significantly enhance neural recovery and prevent permanent sensory neuropathic pain. Therefore, understanding the anatomical landmarks and potential risks during procedures is crucial [28, 31].

Treatment strategies for nerve injuries depend on the severity and type of injury. For lingual nerve injuries, a logical and stepwise approach is recommended for management, with the decision between surgical or nonsurgical treatment strategies being made based on the specific case. In situations involving the inferior alveolar nerve, treatments focus on alleviating symptoms like hyperesthesia and dysesthesia [28]. In summary, nerve damage post-tooth extraction is a complex issue requiring careful consideration from diagnosis to treatment. Understanding the causes, recognizing symptoms early, employing preventive measures, and providing appropriate management are key to minimizing the impact of such injuries and ensuring patient well-being.

#### 7.3.4.1 Inferior Alveolar Nerve

**Anatomical Features and Variation**

The inferior alveolar nerve (IAN), a crucial branch of the mandibular nerve, follows a distinctive path through the mandibular canal in the lower jawbone (Fig. 7.4). Its primary function is to provide sensory innervation to the lower teeth. As the IAN nears the mental foramen, it divides into several terminal branches, including the mental nerve, which exits the mandibular canal and supplies sensation to the lower lip and chin area.

A key aspect of the IAN's anatomical variations includes its relationship with the lower third molar (LM3) roots (Fig. 7.5). The study underlines the heightened risk of nerve injury associated with the position of the IAN relative to these roots, particularly when the nerve is located lingually (toward the tongue side) as opposed to a buccal (cheek side) position [32]. This positional relationship plays a critical role in determining

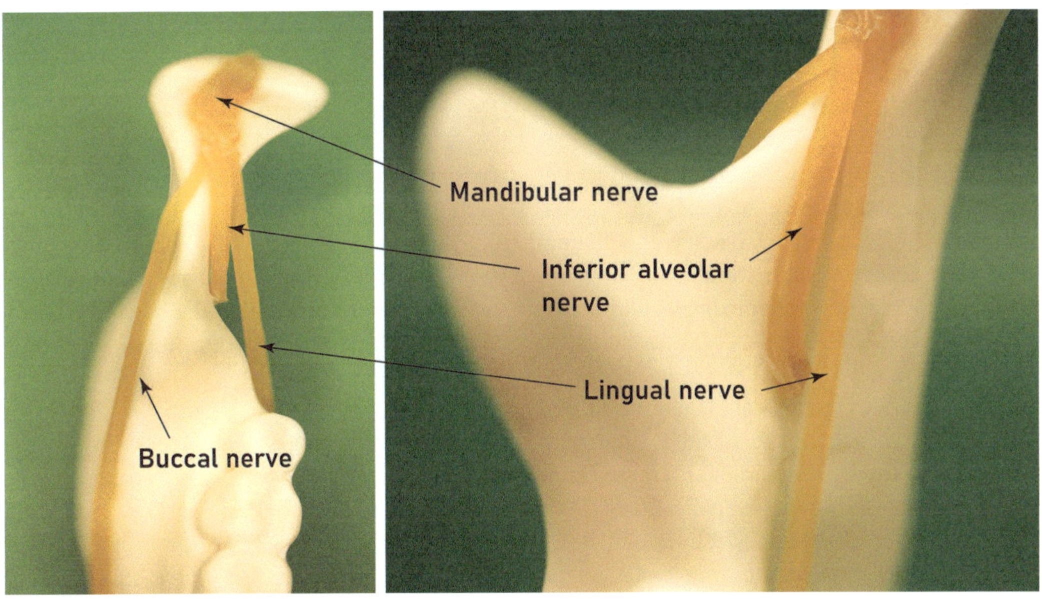


**Fig. 7.4** The anatomical location of the inferior alveolar nerve and other branches from the mandibular nerve

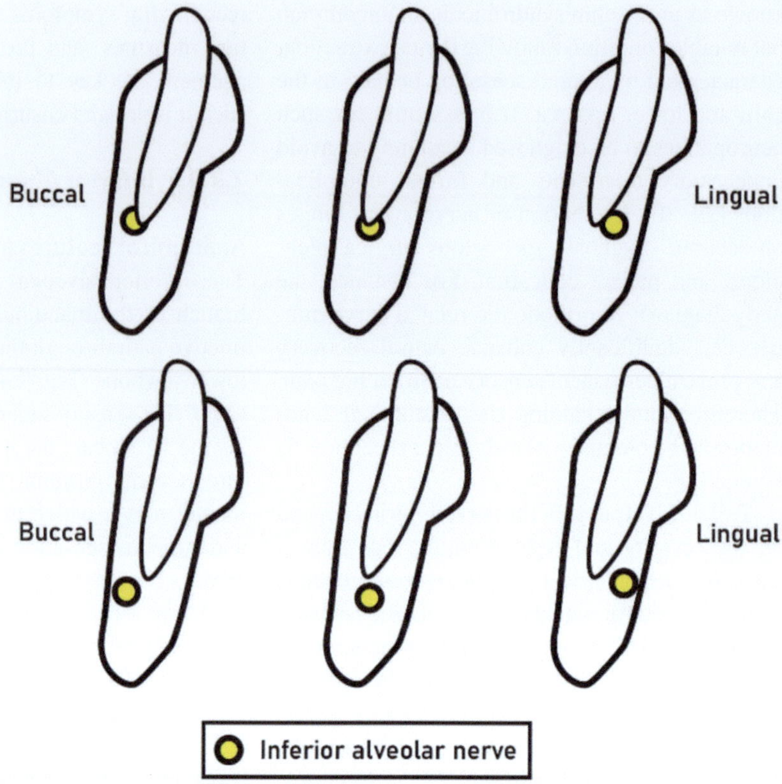


**Fig. 7.5** Relative position of the inferior alveolar nerve to the mandibular third molar

the likelihood of nerve injury during dental procedures, especially in the extraction of third molars.

The anatomical study of 18 human heads revealed several variations in the IAN's structure [33]. Notably, at the entry into the mandibular canal, the IAN forms a plexiform structure by receiving sympathetic branches, which can sometimes impact vegetative ganglion formation. Moreover, in about 16.6% of cases, bridge-like connections between the IAN and the lingual nerve were observed [33], which can be asymmetric and vary in development. Additionally, connections between the IAN and the auriculotemporal nerve were noted. The presence of separate branches from the pre-canalicular portion of the IAN that penetrate the mandible independently is also significant, particularly in the context of mandibular anesthesia application [33].

These detailed anatomical features and variations of the IAN highlight the complexity and the need for careful consideration during dental procedures, especially in extractions and local anesthesia administration, to minimize the risk of nerve injury.

#### Causes of Injury

The systematic review on IAN injury following the removal of impacted mandibular third molars (IMTMs) revealed critical data regarding the prevalence and causes of such injuries. The study identified that out of the total IMTM extractions, 1.20% resulted in transient IAN deficits, while 0.28% led to permanent deficits [34]. This highlights the relative rarity but significant impact of such injuries. The identified risk factors contributing to IAN injury during tooth extraction include the following:

- Depth of impaction: The level at which the IMTM is impacted plays a substantial role in the risk of nerve damage. Teeth impacted deeper within the jaw are more likely to be associated with increased nerve injury risks.
- Proximity to mandibular canal: The risk of IAN injury escalates significantly when the

**Table 7.3** Assessment of inferior alveolar nerve damage

| Category | Test | Description |
|---|---|---|
| Mechanoceptive testing | Contact threshold test | Measures tactile perception threshold using Weinstein–Semmes filaments |
| | Direction test | Assesses ability to identify stimulus direction in a specified area |
| | Two-point discrimination test | Determines the minimum distance between two points perceived as separate |
| Nociceptive testing | Pinprick test | Evaluates pain perception using a small needle |
| | Thermal discrimination test | Test ability to differentiate temperature using acetone-soaked cotton swabs |
| | Current perception threshold test | Measures perception threshold for electrical stimuli |

IMTM is in proximity or directly contacts the mandibular canal, underscoring the importance of preoperative imaging for risk assessment.

- Surgical technique: The surgical approach and techniques employed are pivotal in determining the risk of nerve damage. Certain surgical methods may inherently carry a higher risk of causing IAN injury.
- Intraoperative nerve exposure: Instances where the IAN is exposed during the surgical procedure markedly increase the likelihood of nerve injury, emphasizing the need for meticulous surgical technique.
- Surgeon's experience: The surgeon's experience is a decisive factor in the occurrence of nerve injuries. Surgeons with less experience in such procedures are found to have a higher likelihood of causing nerve damage.

This comprehensive analysis underscores the multifactorial nature of IAN injury risk during IMTM extraction and the need for careful surgical planning and execution.

### Diagnosis

Poort et al. [35] offers comprehensive insights into the methods for diagnosing IAN damage. This study aims to identify practical testing methods suitable for daily clinical practice to grade nerve injury severity and monitor recovery. It reviews various sensory testing methods, including the light touch test with Semmes–Weinstein monofilaments and two-point discrimination tests, highlighting the need for standardized and uniform testing methodology (Table 7.3). The study recommends using the light touch test for grading nerve injury and a visual analog scale-based questionnaire for evaluating subjective sensibility [35]. This approach enables more accurate assessments of IAN injuries and facilitates comparisons across future studies.

Nerve injuries are significant because they can lead to a loss of sensation, motor function, or both, in the affected area. The classification of nerve injuries provides insight into the severity of the injury and the potential for spontaneous recovery or the need for surgical intervention (Fig. 7.6).

- Neuropraxia: This is the mildest form of nerve injury. It involves a temporary disruption of nerve conduction without loss of nerve continuity (Fig. 7.6a). There is a reversible block in nerve conduction leading to a loss of motor function and/or sensation. The classic examples of neuropraxia include "crutch palsy" and "Saturday night palsy," where the injury is due to mechanical pressure causing segmental demyelination. Recovery is typically spontaneous and occurs within days to weeks as the myelin sheath repairs itself (Fig. 7.7).
- Axonotmesis: This injury occurs when the axon is damaged, but the surrounding connective tissue structures, such as the myelin sheath and endoneurial tubes, remain intact (Fig. 7.6b). This leads to Wallerian degeneration and subsequent regeneration of the axon. Recovery depends on the extent of the injury and the distance the axon needs to grow to reconnect with its target; it can take anywhere from 2 to 6 months (Fig. 7.7). The regenera-

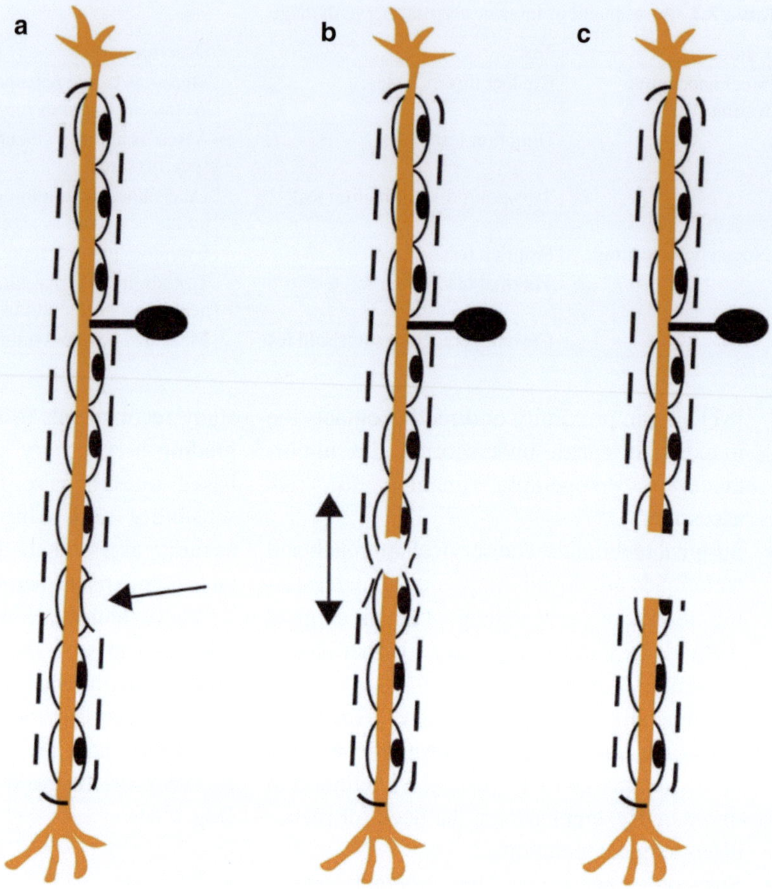


**Fig. 7.6** Classification of nerve injury. (**a**) Neuropraxia, (**b**) axonotmesis, (**c**) neurotmesis

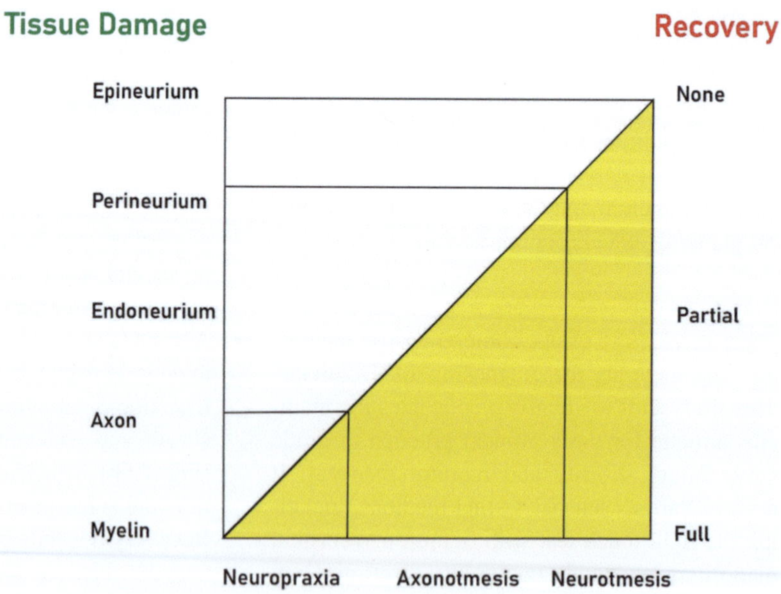


**Fig. 7.7** Relationship among classification of nerve injury, tissue damage, and recovery

tive process is guided by the intact connective tissue structures, which aid in the directionality and success of recovery.

- Neurotmesis: The most severe form of nerve injury, neurotmesis, involves a complete disruption of the nerve and its connective tissue structures (Fig. 7.6c). While originally thought to involve a complete transection of the nerve trunk, severe damage can occur without an actual cut. Recovery is not spontaneous and typically requires surgical intervention. If surgical reconnection is successful, partial recovery may occur within 12 months. However, some cases may result in no recovery due to extensive scarring and disorganization within the nerve, which prevents proper axonal regrowth (Fig. 7.7).

### Treatment

IAN damage is a significant complication associated with the extraction of lower third molars. This condition, often presenting as paresthesia, can profoundly affect a patient's sensory experience and quality of life. Effective management strategies, including both conservative and surgical approaches, are essential for dental professionals to mitigate these complications and promote patient recovery [36].

- Conservative Approaches to IAN Damage
- Conservative management of IAN injury primarily involves monitoring and noninvasive treatments. Monitoring recovery through simple sensory testing is a cornerstone of this approach, allowing clinicians to track the progression of nerve healing and identify patients who may require more intensive intervention [37]. Photobiomodulation (PBM) therapy has emerged as a promising nonsurgical treatment [38]. A study involving 20 patients demonstrated that PBM therapy, using an 808-nm laser, significantly improved sensory recovery compared to conventional treatments like mecobalamine [38]. This suggests that PBM, by reducing pain and inflammation and promoting tissue healing, can be an effective conservative treatment for IAN damage post-extraction. The medications used for managing IAN damage, categorized by their primary action (Table 7.4).
- Surgical Approaches to IAN Damage
- In cases where conservative management is insufficient, surgical interventions may be considered. There is evidence that certain surgical procedures can yield substantial improvements in sensation for patients with IAN damage [37]. However, the decision to proceed with surgery must be weighed against potential risks and the specific circumstances of the injury [36]. Surgical management often requires a nuanced understanding of the types of nerve injuries and their causes, as well as a careful evaluation of the patient's overall prognosis (Fig. 7.8).

**Table 7.4** Medication management for inferior alveolar nerve damage

| Category | Medication type | Examples | Primary use |
|---|---|---|---|
| Anti-inflammatory | Corticosteroids | – | Reducing inflammation and swelling around the nerve |
| | Nonsteroidal anti-inflammatory drugs (NSAIDs) | Ibuprofen | Pain relief and anti-inflammatory effects |
| Neuropsychiatric | Anticonvulsants | Gabapentin, pregabalin | Managing neuropathic pain |
| | Antidepressants | Amitriptyline (tricyclic antidepressant) | Chronic neuropathic pain management |
| | Vitamin supplements | Vitamin B12 (mecobalamine) | Potential nerve repair and regeneration |
| Pain management | Pain relievers | Acetaminophen, prescription painkillers | Direct pain relief |
| Topical agents | Topical anesthetics | Lidocaine | Temporary pain relief in the affected area |

- Decompression: This procedure involves relieving pressure on the nerve. It is typically considered when there is a belief that the nerve is compressed but not completely severed (Fig. 7.8a). Decompression can help in restoring nerve function and reducing symptoms like pain or paresthesia.
- Neurolysis: This involves the removal of scar tissue that may be compressing or entangling the nerve, thus impairing its function (Fig. 7.8b).
- Direct nerve repair (neurorrhaphy): If the nerve is severed but the ends are in good condition and close together, a direct repair may be possible. This involves stitching the nerve ends together (Fig. 7.8c).
- End-to-side neurorrhaphy: In cases where a direct end-to-end repair is not feasible, a connection may be made between the end of the injured nerve and the side of a nearby healthy nerve.
- Nerve Transfer: In some cases, a less critical nerve in the vicinity can be "transferred" to replace the function of the damaged nerve.
- Nerve grafting: In cases where the nerve has been severed or severely damaged, a nerve graft may be necessary. This procedure involves replacing or bridging the damaged section of the nerve with a nerve graft, which can be taken from another part of the patient's body. The goal is to restore as much sensory function as possible (Fig. 7.8d).

The management of IAN injuries, whether conservative or surgical, is marked by a lack of consensus among clinicians, as highlighted by a survey among UK oral health practitioners [39]. This variability in clinical practices, coupled with a general lack of confidence in managing such injuries, underscores the need for standardized treatment guidelines. Developing clear, evidence-based protocols can assist clinicians in making informed decisions about the most appropriate management approach for each patient. It is crucial for dental professionals to understand the advantages and disadvantages of both conservative and surgical approaches. This knowledge

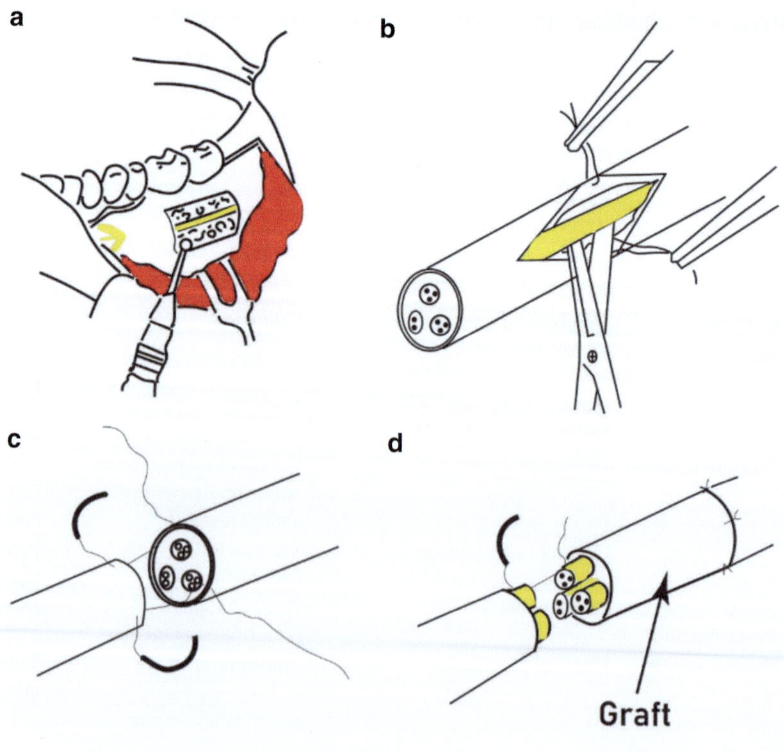


**Fig. 7.8** Surgical management of the inferior alveolar nerve damage. (**a**) Decompression by decortication, (**b**) neurolysis, (**c**) neurorrhaphy, (**d**) nerve graft

enables them to counsel patients effectively about their treatment options, expected outcomes, and the potential timeline for recovery. A comparative analysis, including an algorithm for monitoring and referral, provides a valuable framework for this decision-making process [36].

The treatment of IAN damage following tooth extraction requires a balanced consideration of both conservative and surgical options. Clinicians must continuously assess the severity and progression of nerve injury to determine the most appropriate course of action. With advances in treatments like PBM therapy and a growing understanding of surgical outcomes, there is a pathway toward more effective and patient-centered management of IAN injuries.

#### Prognosis

IAN damage after tooth extraction, especially lower third molar extraction, demonstrates a varying range of recovery rates. A comprehensive literature review indicates that the incidence of IAN injury post-extraction is approximately 0.35–8.4% [40]. A retrospective study of nearly 5000 extractions showed that about 1.1% resulted in IAN impairment, with a higher sensation recovery rate observed within the first 3 months following the injury [41]. Remarkably, about half of the patients showed full recovery after 6 months [41]. This suggests that while IAN injuries can be concerning, a significant proportion of patients experience substantial recovery over time.

Although most IAN injuries are not permanent, the risk of long-term or permanent damage cannot be ignored. Studies suggest that permanent injury, while rare, does occur in a small percentage of cases [36, 42]. The key to mitigating the risk of permanent damage lies in early identification, accurate diagnosis, and prompt, appropriate management of the injury [42].

Several factors influence the prognosis of IAN damage. Age is a notable factor, with older patients (over 24 years old) facing a higher risk of nerve injury and a slower recovery process [40]. The type of impaction, particularly horizontal impactions, is another critical factor that increases the risk of nerve damage. Additionally, extractions performed by less experienced surgeons, such as trainees, may have a higher incidence of associated nerve injuries [40]. The recovery of sensation also tends to be faster in younger patients, and the extent of recovery can vary based on the severity of the initial injury and the timeliness of the treatment [36, 40].

The prognosis of IAN damage after tooth extraction predominantly leans toward recovery, especially with early and appropriate management. However, the potential for permanent damage, albeit low, necessitates a careful approach, including thorough preoperative assessment and skilled surgical technique. Understanding the influencing factors such as patient age, impaction type, and surgeon experience can help in better predicting the outcomes and guiding patients regarding their recovery expectations.

### 7.3.4.2 Lingual Nerve (LN)

#### Anatomical Features and Variation

The lingual nerve is a branch of the posterior division of the mandibular part of the trigeminal nerve. It originates in the infratemporal fossa, situated between the tensor veli palatini and the lateral pterygoid muscle. Here, it is typically joined by the chorda tympani nerve. The LN then proceeds to the floor of the mouth, entering between the mandibular ramus and the medial pterygoid muscle. During its course, the LN may communicate with other nerves such as IAN, auriculotemporal, and mylohyoid nerves. This nerve is responsible for providing general somatic afferent sensation to the anterior two-thirds of the tongue and gingiva. After joining with the chorda tympani, the LN also contributes to the taste sensation of the anterior two-thirds of the tongue [43].

The LN exhibits a wide variation in its pathway from the third molar region to the submandibular gland [43]. It typically travels on the periosteum on the medial surface of the mandible, often positioned opposite the posterior root of the lower third molar (Fig. 7.9). In this area, the nerve is covered only by gingival mucoperi-

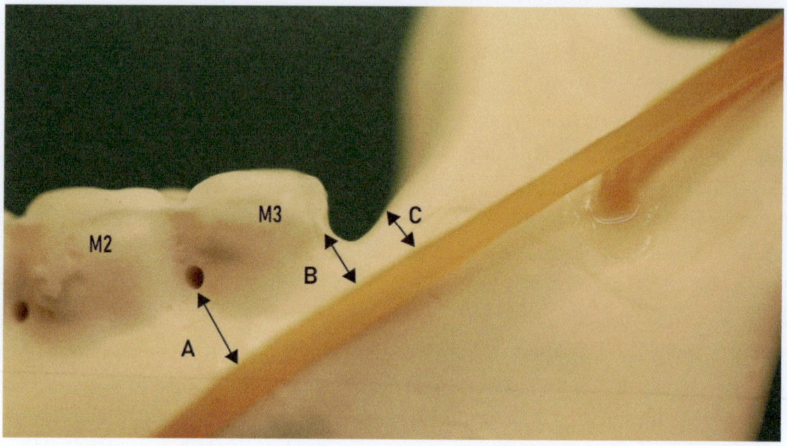


**Fig. 7.9** Distance between lingual nerve and other anatomical landmarks. The shortest distance between mesial surface of third molar (M3) and lingual nerve (A) is 15.5 (8.7~19.9) mm. The shortest distance between distal surface of third molar (M3) and lingual nerve (B) is 9.5 (5.1~16.1) mm. The shortest distance between retromolar region and lingual nerve (C) is 7.8 (3.5~14.2) mm

osteum and is closely bound to the lingual plate of the mandible. Studies have shown that the LN and the lingual cortical plate are in contact 20–62% of the time, while in 4.6–21% of cases, the LN can be located at or above the crest of the bone [43]. Moreover, the LN usually passes lateral to the submandibular duct, moving inferiorly and medially to it on its way to the hyoglossus muscle. In some cadaver studies, the LN was found in a different location, passing above the duct. Additionally, the LN and the IAN typically have a bifurcation located around the mandibular notch. In most cases (66.01%), this bifurcation occurs above the mandibular notch and inferior to the otic ganglion [43].

The understanding of the LN's variable anatomy is crucial due to its proximity to the third molar region, which is a common site for neoplasms, surgeries, and other periodontal operations. The most frequent cause of injury to the LN is during the removal of the mandibular third molar, attributed to its anatomical position and the difficulty in visualizing the LN using computed tomography [43]. This detailed understanding of the LN's course and its anatomical variations is essential for oral and maxillofacial surgeons to minimize the risk of nerve injury during dental procedures, especially those involving the lower third molars.

### Causes of Injury

LN damage during tooth extraction, particularly the extraction of lower third molars (wisdom teeth), can occur due to several factors:

- Anatomical proximity: The LN is near the third molar region. Its variable anatomical course means it may sometimes be positioned near or against the lingual plate of the mandible, making it vulnerable to injury during extraction procedures [43].
- Surgical technique: Improper or aggressive surgical techniques can directly damage the LN. This includes excessive retraction, overextension of surgical flaps, or inadvertent incisions that may cut or compress the nerve.
- Instrumentation: The use of dental instruments like elevators, drills, and extraction forceps can inadvertently traumatize the LN, especially if the nerve is not visualized correctly or if the instruments are used with excessive force near the nerve's location.
- Root removal: The process of removing the roots of the lower third molars, which may be deeply embedded or near the nerve, can put the LN at risk, particularly if the roots are entangled with the nerve fibers.
- Pressure or trauma: The application of pressure or trauma to the mandible during extrac-

tion can cause indirect injury to the LN, such as through stretching, crushing, or contusion.
- Inflammation and swelling: Post-extraction inflammation and swelling can compress the LN, leading to damage.
- Experience of the surgeon: The likelihood of nerve damage can be higher with less-experienced surgeons or in complex cases where the anatomical landmarks are not clearly identifiable.

It is important to note that while LN damage during tooth extraction is a known risk, careful planning, skilled surgical technique, and a thorough understanding of the patient's unique anatomical features can significantly reduce the risk of such an injury. Preoperative imaging, like cone-beam computed tomography (CBCT), can help in identifying the nerve's location relative to the teeth being extracted, thereby aiding in the planning of a safer surgical approach.

**Diagnosis**

The timing of the injury is critical in assessing the type and severity of the nerve injury. Recovery within 4–6 weeks often indicates a neuropraxia-type injury with a good prognosis [28]. More prolonged recovery or improvement over 2–3 months suggests an axonotmesis type injury with variable recovery [28]. No signs of sensory function return beyond 3 months indicate a neurotmesis type injury, associated with a poor prognosis for spontaneous recovery [28].

Physical examination and neurosensory testing involve a detailed history of the injury and current complaints, followed by subjective and objective testing. It helps stratify patients based on the degree of sensory impairment and whether the sensation loss is accompanied by pain. Patients presenting with anesthesia need stratification based on the degree of functional impairment [28].

While the history and physical examination are most important, imaging such as computed tomography (CT) and magnetic resonance imaging (MRI) can be useful. High-resolution MRI and magnetic resonance neurography can offer insights into the condition of the injured nerve, like changes in nerve diameter or position, which may indicate Wallerian degeneration or neuroma formation [28].

**Treatment and Prognosis**

The decision for microsurgical treatment depends on the individual presentation and clinical course. Surgical repair is considered for moderate to severe sensory impairment, dystrophic ageusia, or neuropathic pain of peripheral origin [28]. The time elapsed since the injury is crucial, as the potential for successful repair decreases significantly after 12 months due to Wallerian degeneration and scar tissue formation in the distal nerve segment [28].

For patients with long-standing dysfunctional injury or pain, nonsurgical therapies are the primary mode of treatment. These include behavioral treatments like sensory reeducation and cognitive behavioral therapies, and pharmacologic treatments [28]. Medications used in the acute phase include steroidal anti-inflammatory drugs, narcotic analgesics, and benzodiazepam drugs for anxiety and stress [28]. For chronic neuropathic pain, anticonvulsants and tricyclic antidepressants may be beneficial.

### 7.3.5 Mandibular Fracture After Tooth Extraction

Mandibular fractures following the extraction of lower third molars, though rare, are among the most severe complications of this common oral surgery procedure (Fig. 7.10). These fractures can happen either intraoperatively or as a postoperative complication, typically within the first 4 weeks following surgery [44]. The incidence of these fractures is relatively low, ranging from 0.0034% to 0.075% for lower third molar extractions [44]. Postoperative fractures are more common than intraoperative ones, with incidences reported between 0.0042% to 0.0046% and 0.0033% to 0.0036%, respectively [44].

Mandibular fractures during or after lower third molar extraction can be caused by various factors including inadequate management of surgical instruments, application of excessive force, incorrect surgical techniques, extensive ostectomies,

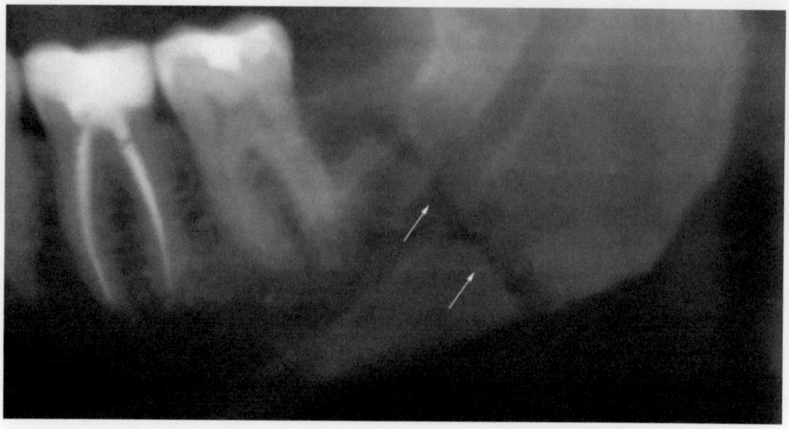

**Fig. 7.10** The mandibular facture 2 weeks after third molar extraction (arrows)

and underestimation of the extraction's difficulty. Pathological bone weakening due to conditions like cystic or malignant injuries, osteoporosis, or medication-related osteonecrosis can also contribute to these fractures. The most vulnerable patients are typically male, over 40 years of age, and the fractures usually occur in the mandibular angle, followed by the body and the canine area [44]. Intraoperative fractures are often attributed to surgical challenges related to the mesioangular position of the third molar and the use of inappropriate surgical instruments like Winter's drift [44].

To minimize the risk of mandibular fractures during or after the extraction of lower third molars, comprehensive preoperative analysis of different risk factors is crucial. This includes considering demographic variables like age and gender, and planning the surgical technique according to the position, angulation, and degree of impaction of the third molar. It is also important to employ proper surgical techniques and conduct a detailed clinical and radiographic evaluation of each case. Intraoperative fractures tend to occur more frequently on the left side of the mandible, whereas postoperative fractures are more common on the right side.

### 7.3.6 Medication-Related Osteonecrosis of the Jaw (MRONJ)

This condition can occur in patients who are taking certain medications like bisphosphonates, typically used for osteoporosis and some cancer treatments (Table 7.5). These medications can interfere with bone turnover, leading to a risk of jawbone necrosis post extraction (Fig. 7.11).

The incidence of MRONJ after tooth extractions can vary widely, ranging between 11% and 50% at MRONJ patient level [45]. MRONJ can occur up to 3 years after the tooth extraction, with risk factors including teeth affected by inflammation before the extraction and additional osteotomy during the surgical procedure [45]. For patients exposed to intravenous (IV) bisphosphonates, the risk of MRONJ after dental extraction has been reported as ranging from 1.6% to 14.8% [46, 47]. This statistic is particularly relevant for patients with cancer treated with IV bisphosphonates. The incidence of MRONJ among patients taking oral bisphosphonates for the management of osteoporosis is significantly lower, generally considered to be between 0.001% and 0.01% [48].

Treatment of MRONJ typically involves a multi-disciplinary approach, focusing on reducing pain, controlling infection of the soft and hard tissues, and minimizing the progression or occurrence of bone necrosis. Strategies may include as follows:

1. Conservative management: This includes the use of oral antimicrobial rinses, systemic antibiotics, and pain management. Conservative management is often the first line of treatment, especially in cases of early-stage MRONJ.

**Table 7.5** Medications associated with medication-related osteonecrosis of the jaw (MRONJ)

| Medication type | Description |
|---|---|
| Bisphosphonates | Primarily used for osteoporosis and bone diseases. Inhibit bone resorption but can impair bone healing |
| Denosumab | A monoclonal antibody for osteoporosis and bone cancers. Inhibits osteoclast formation, affecting bone turnover |
| Antiangiogenic agents | Used in cancer therapy to inhibit new blood vessel formation, which can impair wound healing and jawbone blood supply |
| Immunosuppressants | Increase the risk of MRONJ, especially when combined with drugs like bisphosphonates or denosumab. |
| Corticosteroids | Prolonged use may contribute to MRONJ development, particularly in combination with other high-risk drugs |
| Selective estrogen receptor modulators (SERMs) | Used for osteoporosis treatment. Lower risk compared to bisphosphonates, but still associated with MRONJ |

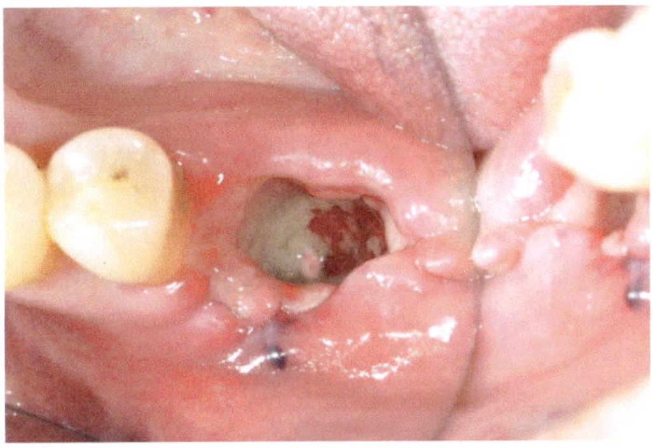

**Fig. 7.11** Medication-related osteonecrosis of the jaw is found after tooth extraction

(a) Medication adjustment: The dosage of the causative medication can be adjusted or discontinued (drug holiday), and an alternative can be administered. This requires consultation with an internist, so a referral should be made for collaborative treatment. Possible medications for MRONJ patients include pentoxifylline and tocopherol. Pentoxifylline is a methylxanthine derivative and a cAMP phosphodiesterase inhibitor. The recommended dosages are 800 mg/day for pentoxifylline and 800 UI/day for tocopherol [49]. Success rates vary according to the literature, with about 70% in Stage 1 and 2, and around 40% in Stage 3 reported.

(b) Improvement in oral hygiene: Maintaining good oral hygiene is crucial to reduce the risk of infection.

(c) Use of antimicrobial mouthwash: Using a mouthwash with antimicrobial properties to limit the number of bacteria in the mouth is also one of the methods to prevent the progression of the disease.

(d) Pain management: As many patients present with pain, especially up to Stage 2, it is often controlled with non-steroidal anti-inflammatory drugs. Proper medication should be administered to manage the patient's pain.

(e) Continuous follow-up: Regular visits for intensive monitoring of the disease's progression are an effective way to prevent its advancement.

2. Surgical intervention: For more advanced cases or when conservative management fails, surgical treatments such as debridement or resection of necrotic bone may be necessary. The goal of surgery is to remove necrotic tissue, reduce bacterial load, and create a stable oral environment.
   (a) Sequestrectomy: Removing the exposed necrotic bone can be an effective way to halt the progression of the disease and alleviate the patient's discomfort.
   (b) Jawbone resection: In more advanced cases, extensive resection of the affected bone can aid in natural healing.
   (c) Pedicled buccal fat flap: Fat tissue, which is rich in blood flow and stem cells, can be used to promote epithelialization of exposed bone following surgical treatment of MRONJ-affected jawbone [50].

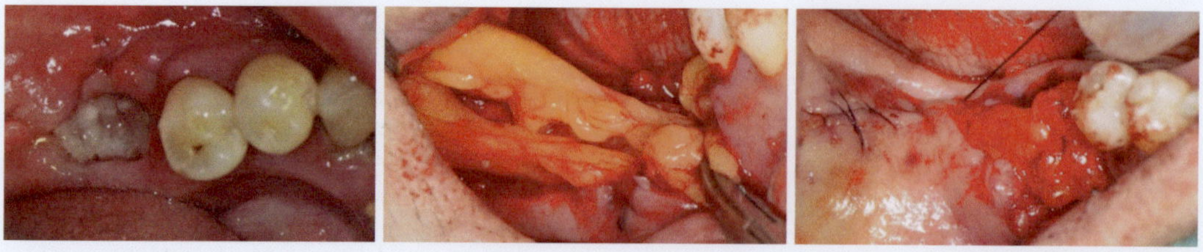

**Fig. 7.12** Surgical management of MRONJ with pedicled buccal fat flap technique. Left panel shows the unhealed extraction socket, characteristic of MRONJ, where healing is impaired due to compromised bone turnover. The area appears inflamed and necrotic, indicating the presence of non-vital bone After performing a sequestrectomy to remove necrotic bone tissue, the pedicled buccal fat flap is carefully raised (middle). The flap is sutured in place, ensuring a snug fit and adequate coverage of the exposed bone (right)

The buccal fat flap can be harvested through an intraoral incision, so no additional incisions are needed beyond those for bone removal (Fig. 7.12). The incision for bone removal can be slightly extended along the anterior vestibule to harvest the flap. The buccal fat, surrounded by a capsule, can be easily brought out by gently teasing it with instruments, being careful not to damage the flap by excessive traction. The harvested buccal fat flap is then carefully applied to the recipient site where the bone was removed, followed by suturing. The area with the transplanted buccal fat flap can heal well and blend naturally with the surrounding tissue. It is important to check the patient's medical history for previous buccal fat flap surgeries, as the volume of available buccal fat may be reduced.

(d) Reconstruction using microvascular flap: Extensive bone removal may necessitate reconstructive surgery [51]. The choice of reconstruction ranges from simple procedures to complex ones requiring microvascular anastomosis, depending on factors such as the extent of the defect and the patient's overall health. In cases of MRONJ-affected jawbone, poor blood supply makes normal wound healing difficult, so free bone grafting is not recommended alone without additional procedures. Microvascular anastomosis can ensure blood supply to the graft, thus increasing the likelihood of successful wound healing, even if the recipient site has poor blood flow. However, jawbone reconstruction using microvascular anastomosis requires prolonged general anesthesia, which may not be suitable for patients with poor overall health.

3. Adjunctive therapies: These may include hyperbaric oxygen therapy, laser therapy, and the use of platelet-rich plasma. However, the effectiveness of these therapies is still under investigation, and they are generally considered adjunctive to the primary treatment modalities.

These statistics underscore the variability in the risk of MRONJ following tooth extraction, heavily influenced by factors such as the type of medication (IV versus oral bisphosphonates) and the preexisting condition of the teeth. Awareness of these risks is crucial for dental surgeons and medical practitioners managing patients who are at risk for or are being treated for osteoporosis or bone metastatic disease.

### 7.3.7 Oroantral Communication (OAC)

This is an abnormal connection between the oral cavity and the maxillary sinus, which can occur after the extraction of upper molars. If not treated properly, it can lead to a chronic sinus infection or a sinusitis. OAC often occurs iatrogenically following the extraction of antral or sinus teeth (Fig. 7.13). The anatomical relationship between

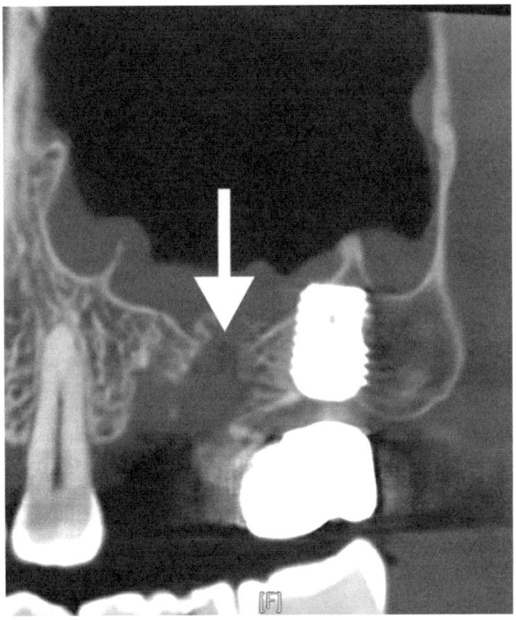

**Fig. 7.13** Oroantral communication after tooth extraction (arrow)

the inferior wall of the maxillary sinus and the maxillary premolar area contributes to this. Sinus effraction can be observed in 3.8–1.3% of cases after maxillary molar extraction. OACs can also result from tumor surgery, implant surgery, trauma, or orthognathic surgery involving the maxilla [52].

Early surgical treatment of OACs is crucial. If left untreated, 50% of patients can develop sinusitis after 48 h, and 90% after 2 weeks [52]. In a healthy sinus, OACs smaller than 5 mm may close spontaneously [52]. However, it is challenging to assess the size of an OAC clinically, necessitating surgical intervention in most cases. Various surgical techniques are available, including the use of surrounding soft tissues like the vestibular flap, palatal flap, or pedicled buccal fat pad (Fig. 7.14). The choice of treatment depends on several factors, including the time of consultation, the presence of associated sinusitis, or the size of the communication. Immediate treatment within 48 h typically involves surgical closure of the OAC [52]. Deferred care may require a two-stage treatment approach. Currently, there is no consensus on the best treatment for OAC. Each technique has its own advantages and disadvantages, and the choice of method must be made on a case-by-case basis, considering all factors regarding the act and the patient. The ideal treatment for OAC should be fast, secure, simple, well-tolerated by patients, cost-effective, and result in good bone and mucosal healing.

### 7.3.8 Dry Socket (Alveolar Osteitis)

Dry socket is characterized by a post-extraction socket with exposed bone that is not covered by a blood clot or healing epithelium. It can persist for days after the extraction procedure. While the clinical techniques for treating dry socket lesions are generally agreed upon, more evidence is needed to conclusively determine the causes. The incidence of dry socket varies, but it is especially prevalent following the extraction of third molars (wisdom teeth), with occurrence rates around 20–30% for these specific extractions [54, 55].

The management of dry socket involves a range of treatments, from rinsing the socket with chlorhexidine or saline to the placement of non-resorbable obtundent dressings and instructions for home rinsing with chlorhexidine. It is noteworthy that a wide array of treatments is in use, indicating a lack of consensus on the most effective approach. The condition remains one of the most examined topics in dentistry, with ongoing research aimed at better understanding and managing it [56].

Understanding the risk factors of dry socket is crucial for identifying high-risk patients, planning treatment, and preparing patients mentally. Some factors, such as the difficulty of the surgery, the surgeon's experience, oral contraception use, and oral hygiene, have shown stronger evidence of being linked to dry socket [57]. However, the influences of other factors like age, gender, and smoking are less clear. Notably, the use of oral contraceptives and its relation to estrogen levels has been suggested as a significant variable in the development of dry socket. It is important to recognize that many risk factors might be a combination of various independent variables, which should be targeted in more comprehensive treatment designs [57].

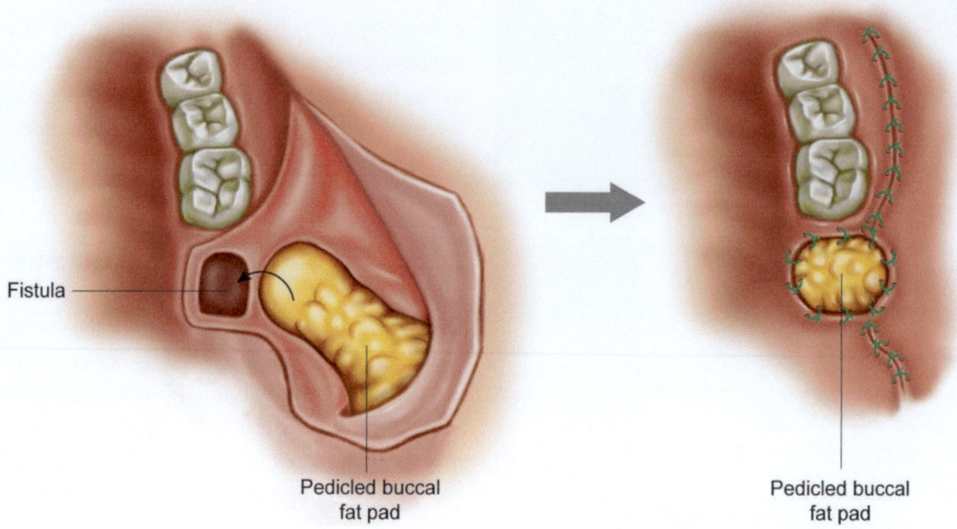


**Fig. 7.14** The utilization of pedicled buccal fat pad in addressing oroantral communication (Adapted from the author's earlier work [53])

### 7.3.9 Trismus

This refers to a restricted ability to open the mouth, often due to injury or inflammation of the muscles and joints near the extraction site. A study focusing on the incidence of trismus following transalveolar extraction of the lower third molar indicated that out of 50 patients, only nine experienced limited mouth opening (MO) during the postoperative period when the duration of the procedure exceeded 30 min. Factors such as pericoronitis and tooth sectioning were contributors. The study also noted that postoperative trismus was more significant in cases of disto-angular impaction [58]. A study evaluating trismus and pain post-extraction investigated whether these responses were related to the difficulty of surgery. The findings suggested that trismus is less severe after simpler extractions (forceps-only) than after more complex surgical extractions. However, the severity of trismus after surgical extraction did not depend on the difficulty of the surgery. Pain, indicated by analgesic use, was also less severe after simpler extractions and tended to decline between days 1 and 5 post-surgery [59]. An investigation focusing on swelling and trismus post-removal of impacted lower third molars by the lingual split technique recorded the duration and pattern of both swelling and trismus. No single cause for these surgical sequelae was identified, underscoring the complexity of factors contributing to postoperative trismus [60].

Trismus typically relieves within 1–2 weeks postoperatively, but in rare cases, it can persist for over a month [61]. A case study reported a patient with trismus at 45 days following mandibular third molar extraction, who received local and systemic anti-inflammatory treatment, combined with incision and drainage therapy [61]. The study also discussed factors associated with the occurrence and development of trismus and management strategies [61]. Another study assessed the effectiveness of combined therapy with corticosteroids and anti-inflammatory analgesics in preventing and reducing trismus after surgical extraction of impacted mandibular third molars [58]. This research, involving 60 patients, concluded that combined therapy was more effective and superior in controlling postoperative trismus compared to individual therapy with either meloxicam (a non-steroidal anti-inflammatory analgesic) or methylprednisolone (a corticosteroid) alone [62].

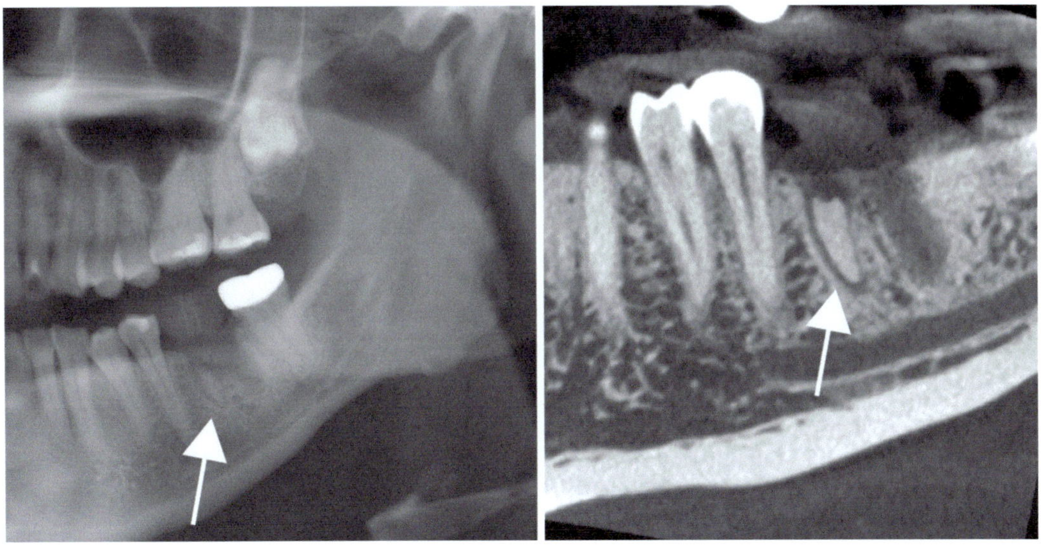

**Fig. 7.15** Panoramic view (left) and subsequent CBCT (right) of a retained mesial root at the first molar extraction site. The panoramic image reveals a radiopaque material at the site of the first molar extraction (arrow). Follow-up CBCT imaging confirms that this material is a retained mesial root of the first molar (arrow). No severe inflammation or bone loss is observed around the retained root

### 7.3.10 Retained Root Tip

Retained root tip after tooth extraction occur due to the fracture of the tooth during extraction. Causes of root fracture include root adhesion, enamel hyperplasia, and severely curved roots. The frequency of root adhesion and enamel hyperplasia tends to be higher in older patients. In the past, it was believed that residual roots smaller than 1 mm do not necessarily need to be removed as they are often absorbed or do not cause other complications. However, considering procedures such as the coronectomy mentioned previously, even residual roots up to 2 mm are unlikely to cause problems if left as is. However, in cases of orthodontic extraction, the presence of residual roots can hinder tooth movement, so they should be completely removed in such cases. Conversely, if the base of the maxillary sinus is close to the root apex, leaving residual roots smaller than 2 mm may be more beneficial for the patient, as removal of these roots could push them into the maxillary sinus. Additionally, it is essential to inform the patient about the presence of residual roots and obtain their understanding. If this process is omitted, the patient may hear about the remaining root during treatment at another dental clinic, making it harder to gain their understanding later. The most advisable approach is to discuss the possibility of residual roots before extraction and obtain consent (Fig. 7.15).

Unlike residual tooth roots, there are cases where the entire tooth remains, which primarily occurs with the lower third molars (Fig. 7.16). This happens when the lingual alveolar bone is thin and adheres to the tooth root, causing the entire tooth to be ejected along with the lingual cortical bone plate during extraction. Preoperative computed tomography can reveal that part of the tooth root protrudes outside the lingual cortical bone plate in such patients. Since extractions are performed using the principle of leverage, if the anatomical structures expected to prevent tooth displacement are weaker than anticipated, the tooth can be ejected in any direction. If this occurs, it is advisable to immediately inform the patient and remove the tooth, but another solution is to wait 2–3 days for hemostasis at the wound site and improved visibility, and then use the incision made during extraction to remove the tooth endoscopically. If the entire tooth has dislodged

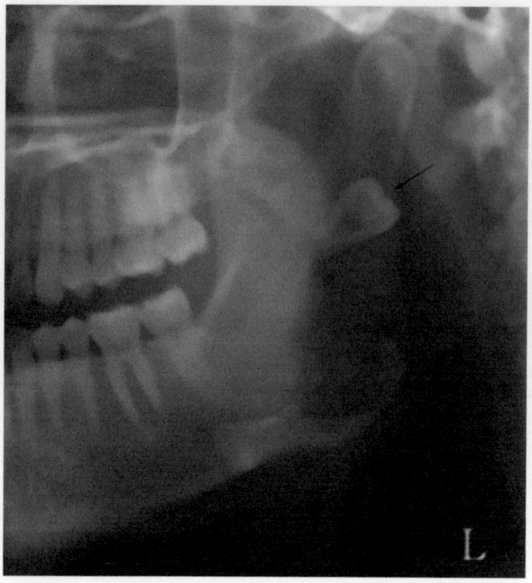

**Fig. 7.16** Displaced mandibular third molar (arrow) during the extraction

into the muscle space, it can be easily removed using an endoscope due to the larger size of the structure to be removed.

## 7.4 Rare But Serious Complications

There have been rare but serious cases of death following tooth extractions reported in the literature, highlighting the importance of recognizing and managing potential complications associated with this common dental procedure. Here are some examples from case reports.

1. Hereditary Angioedema

   A study highlighted hereditary angioedema as a potentially fatal condition that can be triggered by dental treatments, including tooth extraction. In some cases, clinical symptoms such as laryngeal edema, which can lead to asphyxiation, may not manifest for many hours after the procedure [63].
2. Life-Threatening Hemorrhage

   There have been reports of severe postoperative hemorrhages following third molar extractions that resulted in fatal outcomes. This underscores the importance of recognizing the risk of significant bleeding, especially in vulnerable patients or those undergoing complex extractions [64].
3. Uncontrollable Bleeding in Hemophilia Patients

   A case report described two patients with unknown mild hemophilia A who experienced uncontrollable bleeding following tooth extraction. These cases emphasize the importance of thorough preoperative screening for bleeding disorders [17].
4. Rhinocerebral Mucormycosis

   A fatal case of rhinocerebral mucormycosis was reported after dental extractions. This rare but aggressive fungal infection can lead to serious complications, especially in immunocompromised patients [65].

These case reports illustrate that while tooth extractions are generally safe, they are not without risk, particularly in patients with underlying health conditions or in cases where complications like hemorrhage or infection occur. It is crucial for dental professionals to conduct thorough preoperative assessments, use meticulous surgical techniques, and provide comprehensive postoperative care to minimize the risk of such serious complications.

## 7.5 Pre-Extraction Evaluation and Planning

### 7.5.1 Patient Education and Preparation

In the context of tooth extraction, the significance of patient education and preparation cannot be overstated. This process begins from the moment a patient is deemed a candidate for tooth extraction and plays a pivotal role in ensuring a smooth procedure and recovery.

The first step is a comprehensive review of the patient's medical history. This includes an in-depth discussion about any existing medical conditions, medications, allergies, and previous experiences with surgeries or dental procedures. The practitioner must be aware of conditions like diabetes, hypertension, or bleeding disorders, as these can significantly impact the healing process. Additionally, medications such as blood thinners or bisphosphonates require special consideration to avoid complications like excessive bleeding or medication-related osteonecrosis of the jaw.

Once the medical history is reviewed and cleared, the next crucial step is educating the patient about the tooth extraction process. This involves explaining the reasons for extraction, the steps involved in the procedure, and the expected outcomes. It is essential to discuss potential risks and complications, albeit in a manner that does not incite undue anxiety. This transparency helps in building trust and sets realistic expectations for the patient. Preparation for tooth extraction extends beyond the physical aspects; it also includes psychological readiness. Patients often experience anxiety regarding dental procedures, and addressing these concerns is crucial. Techniques such as guided imagery, breathing exercises, or even pharmacological interventions like mild sedatives may be considered to alleviate anxiety.

For the physical preparation, patients should receive clear instructions regarding fasting, if required, and managing routine medications on the day of the procedure. Instructions about arranging transportation post-procedure, especially if sedation is to be used, should be emphasized. Obtaining informed consent is a legal and ethical requirement. This involves ensuring that the patient understands all aspects of the procedure, including potential risks and complications, and can ask questions. Consent should be documented clearly in the patient's records. Finally, ensuring that the patient understands and complies with preoperative instructions is critical. This might include guidelines on oral hygiene, smoking cessation, and adherence to a prescribed preoperative medication regimen. Compliance not only aids in reducing the risk of complications but also enhances the overall success of the procedure.

By thoroughly addressing each of these aspects, healthcare providers can significantly improve the patient experience and outcomes in tooth extraction procedures. This preparatory phase lays the groundwork for a successful extraction and paves the way for a smoother recovery.

### 7.5.2 Techniques to Minimize the Risk of Complications

The successful management of tooth extractions significantly hinges on the meticulous planning and execution of techniques aimed at minimizing the risk of complications. This involves a series of careful considerations and interventions, each tailored to address specific challenges associated with the extraction process. A thorough preoperative assessment is paramount. This includes a detailed dental examination with a focus on the tooth's condition, its position, and its relationship to adjacent anatomical structures. Radiographic evaluations, such as X-rays or CT scans, are crucial for assessing the proximity of the tooth to vital structures like nerves, sinuses, and adjacent teeth (Fig. 7.17). This assessment helps in planning the extraction approach and anticipating potential complications.

In the realm of dental surgery, particularly concerning the extraction of lower third molars, the prediction and prevention of IAN injury is a critical consideration. Two significant studies shed light on the comparative efficacy of CBCT and panoramic radiography (PR) in this context. The study by Reia et al. [66] suggests a superior diagnostic accuracy of CBCT over PR. This research highlights that CBCT exhibits a higher sensitivity (95.1%) in predicting IAN exposure during extraction, compared to PR's sensitivity of 73.9%. Such a high sensitivity rate indicates CBCT's proficiency in accurately identifying cases with potential IAN exposure. In contrast, PR, though having a higher specificity, lacks in sensitivity, indicating its limitation in detecting true positive IAN injury cases. This finding underscores the technological advantage of CBCT, primarily due to its three-dimensional imaging capability, offering a more nuanced and detailed view of the anatomical relationship between the mandibular third molar and the IAN.

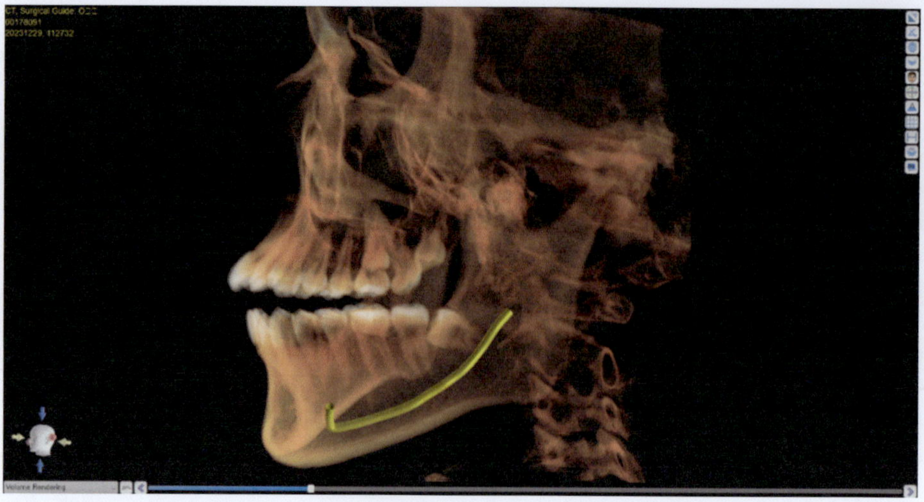

**Fig. 7.17** Tracing the anatomical location of the inferior alveolar nerve using CT scan

However, the study by Liu et al. [67] provides a different perspective, focusing on the diagnostic value of PR. Their meta-analysis reveals a high specificity (0.86) but a lower sensitivity (0.56) for PR in predicting IAN injury [67]. This disparity in sensitivity between the two modalities indicates that while PR is effective in ruling out IAN injury in negative cases, its ability to correctly identify true positive cases of nerve injury is not as reliable. The two-dimensional nature of PR, with its inherent projection-geometric characteristics, is a significant factor contributing to this limitation. It suggests that while PR can be a practical tool for preoperative assessments, especially considering its lower cost and accessibility, its accuracy in predicting IAN injury is not as robust as CBCT.

In summary, the decision to utilize CBCT or PR in predicting IAN injury during lower third molar extraction should be made with careful consideration of these findings. CBCT, with its higher sensitivity, offers a more accurate prediction of IAN exposure, which is crucial for planning and executing safe dental extractions [66]. However, the use of CBCT must be balanced against factors such as its cost, availability, and the patient's exposure to radiation [67]. Despite its limitations in sensitivity, PR remains a valuable tool, particularly in settings where CBCT is not feasible. Ultimately, the choice between these two imaging modalities should be guided by a comprehensive evaluation of each patient's specific situation, weighing the benefits and limitations of both technologies.

Selecting the appropriate surgical instruments and extraction techniques is critical. The choice between a simple extraction and a surgical extraction will depend on factors like tooth visibility, integrity, and root morphology. For teeth with complex root systems or those that are impacted, surgical extractions with careful bone removal and tooth sectioning may be necessary. The use of elevators, forceps, and dental drills should be guided by the specific clinical scenario, aiming for minimal trauma to surrounding tissues. Effective anesthesia management is essential not only for patient comfort but also for reducing the risk of complications. Proper technique in administering local anesthesia ensures adequate pain control and minimizes risks such as needle breakage, infection, or systemic toxicity. The choice of anesthetic agent and the volume administered should be tailored to the patient's medical history and the extent of the procedure.

Minimizing trauma to soft tissues and bone is a critical aspect. Techniques like flap design and gentle tissue retraction are important for providing adequate access while preserving tissue integrity. When bone removal is necessary, careful, and conservative techniques should be employed to avoid unnecessary damage and reduce the risk of postoperative complications such as dry socket or infection. Effective management of bleeding during and post-extraction is vital. This can include local measures like applying pressure, using hemostatic agents, or placing sutures. In patients with bleeding disorders or on anticoagulant therapy, additional precautions and preoperative planning are necessary to manage bleeding risks. Preventing infection starts with strict adherence to aseptic techniques. Sterilization of instruments and the use of barrier methods such as gloves and masks are fundamental. The judicious use of antibiotics, either prophylactically in high-risk patients or therapeutically in cases of postoperative infection, should be based on current clinical guidelines and patient-specific factors.

Postoperative care is a critical component in minimizing complications. Patients should receive clear instructions on wound care, signs of complications, and pain management. Advising patients on proper oral hygiene practices, avoiding smoking, and restricting certain activities helps in promoting healing and preventing issues like infection or alveolar osteitis (dry socket). In conclusion, minimizing the risk of complications in tooth extractions requires a comprehensive approach that encompasses careful preoperative planning, precise execution of the extraction, and diligent postoperative care. By adopting these techniques, dental practitioners can significantly enhance patient outcomes and reduce the incidence of adverse events associated with tooth extraction procedures.

## 7.6 Legal and Ethical Considerations

In the context of dental procedures, particularly tooth extractions, legal and ethical considerations play a pivotal role in ensuring patient welfare and maintaining professional standards. This section delves into three key areas: "Informed Consent and Patient Education," "Handling Complications from a Legal Standpoint," and "Ethical Considerations in Managing Complications."

1. Informed Consent and Patient Education

   Informed consent is a fundamental legal and ethical requirement in dental practice. It involves thoroughly educating the patient about the proposed treatment, including the nature of the procedure, potential risks, alternatives, and expected outcomes. This process should be conducted in a manner that is easily understandable to the patient, considering their age, literacy level, and cultural background. It is crucial that the patient understands not only the procedure itself but also the potential complications and their management. Documentation of informed consent, ideally in the patient's own words, is essential for legal compliance and serves as evidence of the patient's understanding and agreement to the proposed treatment [68].

2. Handling Complications from a Legal Standpoint

   When complications arise during or after a dental procedure, handling them from a legal standpoint requires prompt and appropriate action. This includes acknowledging the complication, informing the patient promptly, and providing necessary corrective treatment. Documentation is key in these scenarios; detailed records of the procedure, the complication, and the steps taken to rectify it are indispensable. In cases where referral to a specialist or additional medical care is required, this should be facilitated without delay. Transparency with the patient and maintaining open communication can often mitigate legal repercussions and helps maintain trust. Additionally, understanding and adhering to local and national regulations and guidelines pertaining to dental practice is crucial in managing such situations legally [69].

3. Ethical Considerations in Managing Complications

   Ethically managing complications goes beyond legal obligations and focuses on the principles of beneficence, non-maleficence, and patient autonomy. Beneficence involves acting in the best interest of the patient, which includes not only treating complications effectively but also taking proactive measures to prevent them. Non-maleficence, or "do no harm," is particularly pertinent in the context of complications—it is essential to avoid actions that could exacerbate the situation and to correct any harm caused because of the dental procedure. Respecting patient autonomy is also critical; this means involving the patient in decision-making processes, especially when dealing with complications and their management. Ethical practice also demands continual self-reflection and learning, ensuring that dental professionals learn from complications to improve practice and patient care [70].

In summary, addressing legal and ethical considerations in tooth extraction and the management of its complications is a multi-faceted process. It requires a comprehensive approach to informed consent and patient education, a legally sound and empathetic approach to managing complications, and an ethical commitment to patient welfare and professional integrity. These elements are integral to fostering trust, ensuring patient safety, and maintaining the highest standards of dental practice.

## 7.7 Conclusion

This chapter has extensively discussed the complexities and challenges involved in the management of tooth extraction complications. We explored various types of complications, ranging from immediate issues like bleeding and pain, to more delayed concerns such as dry socket and infection. Our exploration included not only the clinical aspects but also the preventive measures and treatment strategies to effectively address these complications. Emphasis was placed on the importance of a thorough preoperative assessment, including the assessment of patient history and risk factors, to mitigate the potential for post-extraction problems. Additionally, the role of the dental practitioner in educating patients about postoperative care and the signs of complications was highlighted as a critical component of comprehensive patient care.

The effective management of tooth extraction complications is paramount, not only for patient safety and comfort but also for the long-term success of dental treatments. Complications, if not addressed promptly and effectively, can lead to more significant health issues, including persistent pain, prolonged healing times, and even systemic infections. The role of the dental professional extends beyond the technical execution of the extraction procedure; it encompasses a holistic approach that considers the patient's overall health, effective communication of risks and postoperative care instructions, and readiness to address complications should they arise.

In conclusion, this chapter underscores the necessity of a well-rounded approach to tooth extraction, where prevention, education, and skilled clinical intervention converge to ensure optimal patient outcomes. As the field of dental surgery continues to evolve, the commitment to reducing and managing complications remains a cornerstone of quality patient care and professional excellence in dentistry.

## References


1. Bui CH, Seldin EB, Dodson TB. Types, frequencies, and risk factors for complications after third molar extraction. J Oral Maxillofac Surg. 2003;61:1379–89. https://doi.org/10.1016/j.joms.2003.04.001.
2. Yue Yi EK, Siew Ying AL, Mohan M, Menon RK. Prevalence of postoperative infection after tooth extraction: a retrospective study. Int J Dent. 2021;2021:6664311. https://doi.org/10.1155/2021/6664311.
3. Dallaserra M, Poblete F, Vergara C, et al. Infectious postoperative complications in oral surgery. An observational study. J Clin Exp Dent. 2020;12:e65–70. https://doi.org/10.4317/medoral.55982.
4. Tong DC, Al-Hassiny HH, Ain AB, Broadbent JM. Post-operative complications following dental extractions at the School of Dentistry, University of Otago. N Z Dent J. 2014;110:51–5.
5. Christiaens I, Reychler H. Complications after third molar extractions: retrospective analysis of 1,213 teeth. Rev Stomatol Chir Maxillofac. 2002;103:269–74.
6. Halpern LR, Adams DR. Treatment of medication-related osteonecrosis of the jaw: controversies in causality and therapy. Dent Clin N Am. 2024;68:67–85. https://doi.org/10.1016/j.cden.2023.07.005.
7. Lalla RV, Hodges JS, Treister NS, et al. Tooth-level predictors of tooth loss and exposed bone

after radiation therapy for head and neck cancer. J Am Dent Assoc. 2023;154:519–528.e4. https://doi.org/10.1016/j.adaj.2023.03.009.

8. Biyani P. Complications of tooth extraction. 2020 [cited 2023 Nov 15]. https://www.dentalnotebook.com/complications-tooth-extraction
9. Pei J, Liu J, Chen Y, Liu Y, Liao X, Pan J. Relationship between maxillary posterior molar roots and the maxillary sinus floor: cone-beam computed tomography analysis of a western Chinese population. J Int Med Res. 2020;48:300060520926896. https://doi.org/10.1177/0300060520926896.
10. Mutashar HA, Abdulrazaq SS. Evaluation and comparison of physics forceps and conventional forceps in bilateral dental extraction: a randomized, split-mouth, clinical study. Cureus. 2023;15:e38206. https://doi.org/10.7759/cureus.38206.
11. Matzen LH, Petersen LB, Schropp L, Hermann L, Wenzel A. Risk factors observed in 2-dimensional radiographs for permanent injury of the inferior alveolar nerve after removal of mandibular third molars: a case-control study. Oral Surg Oral Med Oral Pathol Oral Radiol. 2023;136:490–9. https://doi.org/10.1016/j.oooo.2023.05.009.
12. Campana MD, Aliberti A, Acerra A, et al. The effectiveness and safety of autologous platelet concentrates as hemostatic agents after tooth extraction in patients on anticoagulant therapy: a systematic review of randomized, controlled trials. J Clin Med. 2023;12:5342. https://doi.org/10.3390/jcm12165342.
13. Miyazaki R, Sukegawa S, Nakagawa K, et al. Risk factors for delayed-onset infection after mandibular wisdom tooth extractions. Healthcare. 2023;11:871. https://doi.org/10.3390/healthcare11060871.
14. Ono S, Ishimaru M, Yokota I, et al. Risk of post-extraction bleeding with direct oral anticoagulant compared with warfarin: retrospective cohort study using large scale claims data in Japan. Thromb Res. 2023;222:24–30. https://doi.org/10.1016/j.thromres.2022.12.007.
15. Inokoshi M, Kubota K, Yamaga E, Ueda K, Minakuchi S. Postoperative bleeding after dental extraction among elderly patients under anticoagulant therapy. Clin Oral Investig. 2021;25:2363–71. https://doi.org/10.1007/s00784-020-03559-z.
16. Czajkowska S, Rupa-Matysek J, Brzezińska J, Surdacka A, Gil L. Transfusion of fibrinogen concentrate before dental extractions in patients with afibrinogenemia: a narrative review supported by a case report with a proposed treatment protocol. Blood Transfus. 2023;21:168–75. https://doi.org/10.2450/2022.0037-22.
17. Fan G, Shen Y, Cai Y, Zhao JH, Wu Y. Uncontrollable bleeding after tooth extraction from asymptomatic mild hemophilia patients: two case reports. BMC Oral Health. 2022;22:69. https://doi.org/10.1186/s12903-022-02074-9.
18. Mahardawi B, Jiaranuchart S, Rochanavibhata S, Arunjaroensuk S, Mattheos N, Pimkhaokham A. The role of hemostatic agents after tooth extractions: a systematic review and meta-analysis. J Am Dent Assoc. 2023;154:742–752.e1. https://doi.org/10.1016/j.adaj.2023.05.003.
19. Desai S, Berry EJ, Unkel JH, Reinhartz J, Reinhartz D. A case report of haemophilia: a review of haemophilia and oral health implications. Br Dent J. 2023;234:92–5. https://doi.org/10.1038/s41415-023-5448-y.
20. Pierse JE, Dym H, Clarkson E. Diagnosis and management of common postextraction complications. Dent Clin North Am. 2012;56:75–93, viii. https://doi.org/10.1016/j.cden.2011.09.008.
21. Szolnoky G, Szendi-Horváth K, Seres L, Boda K, Kemény L. Manual lymph drainage efficiently reduces postoperative facial swelling and discomfort after removal of impacted third molars. Lymphology. 2007;40:138–42.
22. Domah F, Shah R, Nurmatov UB, Tagiyeva N. The use of low-level laser therapy to reduce postoperative morbidity after third molar surgery: a systematic review and meta-analysis. J Oral Maxillofac Surg. 2021;79:313.e1–313.e19. https://doi.org/10.1016/j.joms.2020.09.018.
23. Lodi G, Azzi L, Varoni EM, et al. Antibiotics to prevent complications following tooth extractions. Cochrane Database Syst Rev. 2021;2:CD003811. https://doi.org/10.1002/14651858.CD003811.pub3.
24. Koray M, Ofluoglu D, Onal EA, et al. Efficacy of hyaluronic acid spray on swelling, pain, and trismus after surgical extraction of impacted mandibular third molars. Int J Oral Maxillofac Surg. 2014;43:1399–403. https://doi.org/10.1016/j.ijom.2014.05.003.
25. Rana M, Gellrich NC, Ghassemi A, Gerressen M, Riediger D, Modabber A. Three-dimensional evaluation of postoperative swelling after third molar surgery using 2 different cooling therapy methods: a randomized observer-blind prospective study. J Oral Maxillofac Surg. 2011;69:2092–8. https://doi.org/10.1016/j.joms.2010.12.038.
26. Sukegawa S, Yokota K, Kanno T, et al. What are the risk factors for postoperative infections of third molar extraction surgery: a retrospective clinical study? Med Oral Patol Oral Cir Bucal. 2019;24:e123–9. https://doi.org/10.4317/medoral.22556.
27. Caniff KE, Young LR, Truong S, et al. Postextraction infection and antibiotic prescribing among veterans receiving dental extractions. Infect Control Hosp Epidemiol. 2021;42:1431–6. https://doi.org/10.1017/ice.2021.15.
28. Romsa B, Ruggiero SL. Diagnosis and management of lingual nerve injuries. Oral Maxillofac Surg Clin North Am. 2021;33:239–48. https://doi.org/10.1016/j.coms.2020.12.006.
29. Jadun S, Miller D, Renton T. Orthodontic-related nerve injuries: a review and case series. Br Dent J. 2020;229:244–8. https://doi.org/10.1038/s41415-020-1994-8.
30. Clauser B, Barone R, Briccoli L, Baleani A. Complications in surgical removal of mandibular third molars. Minerva Stomatol. 2009;58:359–66.

31. Elahi F, Manolitsis N, Ranganath YS, Reddy C. Mental nerve neuropathy following dental extraction. Pain Physician. 2014;17:E375–80.
32. Li Y, Ling Z, Zhang H, et al. Association of the inferior alveolar nerve position and nerve injury: a systematic review and meta-analysis. Healthcare. 2022;10:1782. https://doi.org/10.3390/healthcare10091782.
33. Rácz L, Maros T, Seres-Sturm L. Die anatomischen Variationen des Nervus alveolaris inferior und ihre Bedeutung in der Praxis. Anat Anz. 1981;149:329–32.
34. Kang F, Sah MK, Fei G. Determining the risk relationship associated with inferior alveolar nerve injury following removal of mandibular third molar teeth: a systematic review. J Stomatol Oral Maxillofac Surg. 2020;121:63–9. https://doi.org/10.1016/j.jormas.2019.06.010.
35. Poort LJ, van Neck JW, van der Wal KG. Sensory testing of inferior alveolar nerve injuries: a review of methods used in prospective studies. J Oral Maxillofac Surg. 2009;67:292–300. https://doi.org/10.1016/j.joms.2008.06.076.
36. Mahon N, Stassen LF. Post-extraction inferior alveolar nerve neurosensory disturbances--a guide to their evaluation and practical management. J Ir Dent Assoc. 2014;60:241–50.
37. Robinson PP, Loescher AR, Yates JM, Smith KG. Current management of damage to the inferior alveolar and lingual nerves as a result of removal of third molars. Br J Oral Maxillofac Surg. 2004;42:285–92. https://doi.org/10.1016/j.bjoms.2004.02.024.
38. Qi W, Wang Y, Huang YY, et al. Photobiomodulation therapy for management of inferior alveolar nerve injury post-extraction of impacted lower third molars. Lasers Dent Sci. 2020;4:25–32. https://doi.org/10.1007/s41547-019-00075-6.
39. Orchard A, Adatia A, Moore R, Prabhu S. Management of inferior alveolar nerve and lingual nerve injuries in the UK - a cross-sectional study. Br J Oral Maxillofac Surg. 2022;60:927–32. https://doi.org/10.1016/j.bjoms.2022.01.012.
40. Sarikov R, Juodzbalys G. Inferior alveolar nerve injury after mandibular third molar extraction: a literature review. J Oral Maxillofac Res. 2014;5:e1. https://doi.org/10.5037/jomr.2014.5401.
41. Queral-Godoy E, Valmaseda-Castellón E, Berini-Aytés L, Gay-Escoda C. Incidence and evolution of inferior alveolar nerve lesions following lower third molar extraction. Oral Surg Oral Med Oral Pathol Oral Radiol Endod. 2005;99:259–64. https://doi.org/10.1016/j.tripleo.2004.06.001.
42. Cade TA. Paresthesia of the inferior alveolar nerve following the extraction of the mandibular third molars: a literature review of its causes, treatment, and prognosis. Mil Med. 1992;157:389–92.
43. Ostrowski P, Bonczar M, Wilk J, et al. The complete anatomy of the lingual nerve: a meta-analysis with implications for oral and maxillofacial surgery. Clin Anat. 2023;36:905–14. https://doi.org/10.1002/ca.24033.
44. Guillaumet-Claure MA, Juiz-Camps AM, Gay-Escoda C. Prevalence of intraoperative and postoperative iatrogenic mandibular fractures after lower third molar extraction: a systematic review. J Clin Exp Dent. 2022;14:e85–94. https://doi.org/10.4317/jced.58390.
45. Schwech N, Nilsson J, Gabre P. Incidence and risk factors for medication-related osteonecrosis after tooth extraction in cancer patients-a systematic review. Clin Exp Dent Res. 2023;9:55–65. https://doi.org/10.1002/cre2.698.
46. Sandhu S, Salous MH, Sankar V, Margalit DN, Villa A. Osteonecrosis of the jaw and dental extractions: a single-center experience. Oral Surg Oral Med Oral Pathol Oral Radiol. 2020;130:515–21. https://doi.org/10.1016/j.oooo.2020.07.001.
47. Muthukrishnan A, Bijai Kumar L, Ramalingam G. Medication-related osteonecrosis of the jaw: a dentist's nightmare. BMJ Case Rep. 2016;2016:bcr2016214626. https://doi.org/10.1136/bcr-2016-214626.
48. FitzGerald P. American dental association guidelines for management of osteonecrosis of the jaw. 2019 [cited 2023 Nov 15]. https://americanbonehealth.org/osteoporosis/american-dental-association-guidelines-for-management-of-osteonecrosis-of-the-jaw
49. Cavalcante RC, Tomasetti G. Pentoxifylline and tocopherol protocol to treat medication-related osteonecrosis of the jaw: a systematic literature review. J Craniomaxillofac Surg. 2020;48(11):1080–6. https://doi.org/10.1016/j.jcms.2020.09.008.
50. Rotaru H, Kim MK, Kim SG, Park YW. Pedicled buccal fat pad flap as a reliable surgical strategy for the treatment of medication-related osteonecrosis of the jaw. J Oral Maxillofac Surg. 2015;73(3):437–42. https://doi.org/10.1016/j.joms.2014.09.023.
51. Oh H, Kwon D, Ahn J, Paeng JY. Reconstruction of mandibular defects in osteoradionecrosis and medication-related osteonecrosis of the jaw using fibula free flap and management of postoperative wound infections. Maxillofac Plast Reconstr Surg. 2022;44:37. https://doi.org/10.1186/s40902-022-00366-2.
52. Konate M, Sarfi D, El Bouhairi M, Benyahya I. Management of oroantral fistulae and communications: our recommendations for routine practice. Case Rep Dent. 2021;2021:7592253. https://doi.org/10.1155/2021/7592253.
53. Kim MK, Han W, Kim SG. The use of the buccal fat pad flap for oral reconstruction. Maxillofac Plast Reconstr Surg. 2017;39:5. https://doi.org/10.1186/s40902-017-0105-5.
54. Mamoun J. Dry socket etiology, diagnosis, and clinical treatment techniques. J Korean Assoc Oral Maxillofac Surg. 2018;44:52–8. https://doi.org/10.5125/jkaoms.2018.44.2.52.
55. Torres-Lagares D, Serrera-Figallo MA, Romero-Ruíz MM, Infante-Cossío P, García-Calderón M,

Gutiérrez-Pérez JL. Update on dry socket: a review of the literature. Med Oral Patol Oral Cir Bucal. 2005;10(81–85):77–81.

56. Bowe DC, Rogers S, Stassen LF. The management of dry socket/alveolar osteitis. J Ir Dent Assoc. 2011–2012;57:305–10.
57. Rakhshan V. Common risk factors of dry socket (alveolitis osteitis) following dental extraction: a brief narrative review. J Stomatol Oral Maxillofac Surg. 2018;119:407–11. https://doi.org/10.1016/j.jormas.2018.04.011.
58. Balakrishnan G, Narendar R, Kavin T, Venkataraman S, Gokulanathan S. Incidence of trismus in transalveolar extraction of lower third molar. J Pharm Bioallied Sci. 2017;9(Suppl 1):S222–7. https://doi.org/10.4103/jpbs.JPBS_161_17.
59. Garcia Garcia A, Gude Sampedro F, Gandara Rey J, Gallas Torreira M. Trismus and pain after removal of impacted lower third molars. J Oral Maxillofac Surg. 1997;55:1223–6. https://doi.org/10.1016/s0278-2391(97)90172-5.
60. Rood JP, Yates C, Buchanan M. Postoperative swelling and trismus after mandibular third molar removal with the lingual split bone technique. Int J Oral Surg. 1979;8:31–5. https://doi.org/10.1016/s0300-9785(79)80036-8.
61. Zhang Y, Zhuang P, Jia B, et al. Persistent trismus following mandibular third molar extraction and its management: a case report and literature review. World Acad Sci J. 2021;3:2. https://doi.org/10.3892/wasj.2020.73.
62. Selimović E, Ibrahimagić-Šeper L, Šišić I, Sivić S, Huseinagić S. Prevention of trismus with different pharmacological therapies after surgical extraction of impacted mandibular third molar. Med Glas. 2017;14(1):145–51. https://doi.org/10.17392/871-16.
63. Viciano J, D'Anastasio R, D'Ovidio C, Costantini S, Carnevale A, Capasso L. Estimation of date of death through wound healing of an extraction socket: a case report. Forensic Sci Int. 2017;275:e6–e11. https://doi.org/10.1016/j.forsciint.2017.03.008.
64. Moghadam HG, Caminiti MF. Life-threatening hemorrhage after extraction of third molars: case report and management protocol. J Can Dent Assoc. 2002;68:670–4.
65. Kim J, Fortson JK, Cook HE. A fatal outcome from rhinocerebral mucormycosis after dental extractions: a case report. J Oral Maxillofac Surg. 2001;59:693–7. https://doi.org/10.1053/joms.2001.23407.
66. Reia VCB, de Toledo Telles-Araujo G, Peralta-Mamani M, Biancardi MR, Rubira CMF, Rubira-Bullen IRF. Diagnostic accuracy of CBCT compared to panoramic radiography in predicting IAN exposure: a systematic review and meta-analysis. Clin Oral Investig. 2021;25:4721–33. https://doi.org/10.1007/s00784-021-03942-4.
67. Liu W, Yin W, Zhang R, Li J, Zheng Y. Diagnostic value of panoramic radiography in predicting inferior alveolar nerve injury after mandibular third molar extraction: a meta-analysis. Aust Dent J. 2015;60:233–9. https://doi.org/10.1111/adj.12326.
68. Ferrús-Torres E, Valmaseda-Castellón E, Berini-Aytés L, Gay-Escoda C. Informed consent in oral surgery: the value of written information. J Oral Maxillofac Surg. 2011;69:54–8. https://doi.org/10.1016/j.joms.2010.05.036.
69. Curley AW. The law and dentoalveolar complications: trends and controversies. Oral Maxillofac Surg Clin North Am. 2011;23:475–84. https://doi.org/10.1016/j.coms.2011.04.003.
70. Owsiany DJ. The intersection of dental ethics and law. J Am Coll Dent. 2008;75:47–54.

# 8 Extraction in Medically Compromised Patients

## Contents



## 8.1 Introduction

Tooth extraction is a routine dental procedure that may present significant challenges for medically compromised patients. It is essential to comprehend how medical conditions can impact dental extractions to ensure the safety and well-being of these individuals. Various medical conditions can influence the approach, anesthesia choice, and postoperative care in tooth extraction procedures.

In cases where patients have cardiovascular conditions such as high blood pressure or heart disease, special considerations must be taken [1]. The stress associated with tooth extraction can cause an increase in blood pressure, potentially leading to complications. In such cases, it may be necessary to coordinate with the patient's cardiologist and adjust the anesthesia and medication regimen accordingly to minimize risks.

Patients with bleeding disorders, such as hemophilia or those taking anticoagulant medications, need careful management during tooth extractions. These individuals are at an increased risk of excessive bleeding during and after the procedure [2–4]. Comprehensive preoperative evaluation, including coagulation assessments, is crucial for determining the appropriate hemostatic measures, such as discontinuing medication or adjusting dosages, to minimize bleeding risks.



S.-G. Kim et al., *Advanced Strategies for Tooth Extraction in Dentistry*,
https://doi.org/10.1007/978-981-97-6532-4_8

Patients with diabetes have unique oral health challenges, as the disease can lead to periodontal disease and compromised wound healing [5]. Dentists must exercise caution in managing blood glucose levels, as well as closely monitor any potential oral infections in these patients.

Similarly, patients with compromised immune systems, such as those undergoing chemotherapy or organ transplant recipients, require specialized care during tooth extraction. These individuals have an increased susceptibility to infections, and postoperative healing may be delayed [6–8]. Close coordination with the patient's oncologist or transplant team is imperative to ensure that appropriate precautions are taken, including the use of prophylactic antibiotics and close monitoring for signs of infection.

In conclusion, understanding the implications of medical conditions in dental settings is paramount to ensuring the safety and well-being of medically compromised patients undergoing tooth extraction. Considerations must be taken with respect to cardiovascular conditions, bleeding disorders, diabetes, and compromised immune systems. By adapting the approach, anesthesia choice, and postoperative care, dental professionals can mitigate potential risks and provide optimal treatment outcomes for these patients.

## 8.2 Preoperative Assessment

1. Medical History and Evaluation

   The cornerstone of preoperative assessment in medically compromised patients is a thorough medical history. This step is critical for identifying any underlying health conditions that could affect the course of the dental procedure. A comprehensive medical history should include details about current and past illnesses, hospitalizations, ongoing treatments, medications, allergies, and any previous experiences with anesthesia or surgeries. This information helps in creating a holistic picture of the patient's health status and in anticipating potential complications during the extraction procedure.

   An essential part of the preoperative assessment is to identify any "red flags" in the patient's medical history that might contraindicate tooth extraction or require special precautions. These include, but are not limited to, conditions like uncontrolled diabetes, recent myocardial infarction, bleeding disorders, or use of medications such as anticoagulants that can affect clotting. Recognizing these factors is crucial for ensuring patient safety and for deciding whether the extraction can be safely performed or if alternative treatments should be considered.

2. Interdisciplinary Collaboration

   In the context of treating medically compromised patients, the role of interdisciplinary collaboration becomes paramount. Dental professionals often need to work closely with a range of medical professionals to ensure comprehensive and safe patient care. This collaboration involves sharing patient information, understanding the implications of medical conditions on dental procedures, and formulating a treatment plan that considers the patient's overall health. Such teamwork is essential for minimizing risks and optimizing outcomes in dental extractions for medically compromised patients.

   Coordinating care with a patient's primary physician and other relevant specialists is a critical component of the preoperative assessment. This coordination ensures that the dentist is aware of the patient's current medical treatments and any advice or precautions from their healthcare providers. It may involve discussing the patient's health status, reviewing medications, and determining any necessary adjustments before the dental procedure. Effective communication between dentists, primary care physicians, and specialists is vital for a unified approach to patient care, particularly in complex cases where multiple health issues are present.

3. Risk Assessment and Management

   Effective preoperative assessment involves a detailed analysis of the patient's risk levels. This assessment is not just about identifying existing medical conditions, but also about categorizing these risks in terms of their potential impact on the dental extraction procedure. Risk categorization may range from low to high, based on factors such as the severity and stability of the medical condition, the complexity of the planned dental procedure, and the patient's overall health status. This step is crucial for making informed decisions about the feasibility and safety of performing an extraction and for planning the procedure accordingly.

Once the risks are identified and categorized, the next step is to develop strategies for risk mitigation. This involves tailoring the dental treatment plan to minimize potential complications. Strategies may include modifying the surgical technique, adjusting anesthesia, preparing for emergency management, and scheduling post-operative monitoring. In some cases, it might also involve deferring the extraction until medical conditions are better controlled or stabilized. The goal is to proactively address potential problems, ensuring the safest possible outcome for the patient.

## 8.3 Specific Medical Conditions and Considerations

### 8.3.1 Cardiovascular Diseases

Patients with cardiovascular diseases such as hypertension and heart failure require special consideration during dental procedures, including tooth extractions [1]. The primary concern is to manage these conditions to prevent any cardiac complications during and after the dental treatment. In managing patients with hypertension, it is essential to monitor and evaluate their blood pressure to ensure it falls within a safe range for dental procedures. Generally, a systolic blood pressure below 180 mmHg and a diastolic pressure below 110 mmHg are considered acceptable for routine dental treatments [9]. However, these thresholds may vary based on individual patient circumstances and should be evaluated in conjunction with the patient's overall cardiovascular health and history. For those with heart failure, the stability of their condition should be assessed, and any signs of decompensated heart failure should be addressed before proceeding with dental treatments. It is also crucial to coordinate with the patient's cardiologist or healthcare provider to ensure that their cardiovascular condition is optimally managed and stable before undergoing dental extractions.

For patients with heart failure, the severity and stability of their condition must be carefully evaluated before proceeding with dental treatments like extractions. Heart failure can be categorized based on functional capacity and objective evidence of the severity of the condition [10]. For instance:

- Mild heart failure (NYHA Class I): Patients with no limitation of physical activity. Ordinary physical activity does not cause undue fatigue, palpitation, or dyspnea (shortness of breath).
- Moderate heart failure (NYHA Class II or III): Patients with slight (Class II) or marked (Class III) limitation of physical activity. They are comfortable at rest, but ordinary physical activity results in fatigue, palpitation, or dyspnea.
- Severe heart failure (NYHA Class IV): Patients with inability to carry on any physical activity without discomfort. Symptoms of heart failure are present even at rest, with increased discomfort with any physical activity.

Patients with mild heart failure may often proceed with dental treatments with standard precautions. However, those in the moderate to severe categories, especially NYHA Class III and IV, may require additional assessment and stabilization. In cases of severe heart failure, elective dental procedures should generally be deferred until the patient's condition is optimally managed and stable, often in collaboration with their cardiologist or healthcare provider.

When dealing with patients on anticoagulant therapy, careful planning is needed to balance the risk of bleeding during dental procedures with the risk of thromboembolic events due to altering anticoagulant medication [3, 4]. The concept of a "drug holiday," where anticoagulant medication is temporarily discontinued, may be considered. However, this decision should always be made in close consultation with the patient's cardiologist or primary care physician, based on the patient's individual risk factors.

Before proceeding with dental extractions, it is important to conduct relevant lab tests to assess the patient's coagulation status [11]. The most common tests include:

- INR (International Normalized Ratio): For patients on warfarin, an INR level typically needs to be within a certain therapeutic range, usually between 2.0 and 3.0 for most indications, but this can vary based on individual circumstances [12].
- Platelet function tests: For those on antiplatelet medications, like aspirin or clopidogrel.
- Direct oral anticoagulant (DOAC) levels: For patients on newer anticoagulants, such as dabigatran, rivaroxaban, or apixaban.

The timing of the drug holiday, if considered appropriate, and the timing of the lab tests should be carefully planned to align with the scheduled dental procedure. The anticoagulant therapy is usually resumed as soon as it is clinically safe to do so post-procedure, to minimize the risk of thromboembolic complications.

### 8.3.2 Diabetes Mellitus

Managing diabetic patients undergoing dental extractions requires special precautions due to their altered healing response and increased risk of infection [5]. It is important to ensure that their diabetes is well-controlled prior to the procedure. This can involve:

- Reviewing recent blood glucose levels: Ensuring that the patient's blood sugar is within an acceptable range reduces the risk of postoperative complications.
- Consulting with the patient's endocrinologist or primary care physician: This helps in understanding the patient's diabetic control and any adjustments needed in their diabetic medication around the time of surgery.
- Timing of the procedure: Ideally, dental extractions in diabetic patients should be scheduled for a time when the patient's blood sugar levels are most stable, often in the morning.
- Preoperative blood sugar testing: This helps to ensure the patient is in a good metabolic state before the procedure. There are general guidelines regarding preoperative blood sugar levels that, if exceeded, may warrant postponing a tooth extraction or other elective dental procedures in diabetic patients. These guidelines are based on the need to minimize the risk of complications such as poor wound healing and increased risk of infection. A common threshold is a fasting blood glucose level of <180 mg/dL (10 mmol/L) [13]. Levels above this may indicate poorly controlled diabetes, increasing the risk of postoperative complications. An HbA1c level is often used to assess long-term glycemic control. While the specific cutoff can vary, an HbA1c level >8–9% might suggest poor diabetes control. Some practitioners might use a more conservative threshold, such as 7%, especially in procedures with higher risk of complications [14, 15].

In addition, specific considerations should be given to wound healing in diabetic patients. Enhanced oral hygiene, possibly including antiseptic mouth rinses, and close follow-up to monitor for signs of infection or delayed healing are recommended.

### 8.3.3 Immunocompromised Patients

Patients who are immunocompromised, such as those with HIV, organ transplant recipients, or undergoing chemotherapy, present unique challenges in dental care, particularly in procedures like tooth extraction. These patients are at an increased risk of infections and may have a compromised healing process [6–8, 16]. Dental procedures in these patients require careful consideration, often involving consultation with their medical team, and may necessitate additional prophylactic measures to prevent infection.

Infection control and promoting healing are paramount in managing immunocompromised patients undergoing dental extractions. This involves employing strict aseptic techniques, which entail rigorous infection control measures in the dental office to prevent postoperative infections. Additionally, postoperative care is crucial, involving closely monitoring for any signs of infection or delayed healing. This may include more frequent follow-ups and detailed postoperative instructions tailored to the patient's specific immune status. Patient education is also essential in managing immunocompromised patients undergoing dental extractions. This includes educating patients about signs of infection, emphasizing the importance of maintaining oral hygiene, and instructing them on when to seek immediate medical attention post-procedure.

### 8.3.4 Other Conditions

1. Renal disease, respiratory disorders, osteoporosis, etc.

   This subsection addresses a range of other significant medical conditions that can impact dental extraction procedures, each requiring specific considerations.

   (a) Renal disease [17, 18]: Patients with renal disease, particularly those on dialysis, have an altered ability to metabolize and excrete drugs, which can affect anesthesia and pain management. They also have an increased risk of bleeding and infection. Coordination with the patient's nephrologist for optimal timing of the procedure, especially in relation to dialysis sessions, is crucial.

   (b) Respiratory disorders: Conditions such as chronic obstructive pulmonary disease (COPD) and asthma can affect a patient's ability to tolerate certain dental procedures and anesthesia [19]. Preoperative assessment should include a review of the patient's current respiratory status and medication regimen. Modifications in the dental procedure, including anesthesia, may be necessary to minimize respiratory stress.

   (c) Osteoporosis: Patients taking medications for osteoporosis, particularly bisphosphonates, are at risk for osteonecrosis of the jaw following dental extractions [20]. It is important to review the patient's medication history, and in some cases, consultation with the patient's endocrinologist or primary care physician may be warranted. The decision to proceed with extraction should be made carefully, weighing the risks and benefits.

2. Specific considerations for each condition

   Each of these conditions necessitates a unique approach to dental care:

   (a) Renal disease: Adjustments in medication types and dosages may be required. Precautions to minimize bleeding and infection risks are essential.

   (b) Respiratory disorders: Ensuring a stress-free environment, possibly using supplemental oxygen during the procedure, and avoiding certain sedatives can help manage patients with respiratory disorders.

   (c) Osteoporosis: A thorough review of the patient's medication, especially the duration of bisphosphonate therapy, is essential. In some cases, a "drug holiday" may be considered, but this decision should be made in collaboration with the patient's healthcare provider.

For all these conditions, a multidisciplinary approach involving the patient's primary care physician and specialists is critical to ensure safe and effective dental treatment.

## 8.4 Surgical Techniques and Modifications

1. Modifying Surgical Approaches

   In treating medically compromised patients, it is often necessary to modify standard surgical approaches to accommodate their specific health needs. This may include altering the traditional methods of tooth extraction to reduce stress on the patient, minimize the risk of complications, and ensure a smoother recovery. For example, in patients with cardiovascular disease, techniques that reduce the duration of surgery and limit excessive bleeding are preferred.

Minimally invasive surgical techniques are particularly beneficial for medically compromised patients. These techniques typically involve smaller incisions, less tissue manipulation, and reduced trauma to the surgical site. Such approaches can lead to decreased postoperative pain, lower risk of complications, and faster healing. Examples include flapless extractions, laser-assisted procedures, or piezoelectric surgery. These methods are especially advantageous in patients with conditions like diabetes, where healing might be impaired, or in immunocompromised patients to reduce the risk of infection.

2. Anesthesia and Sedation

   Selecting the right type of anesthesia and sedation is critical in managing medically compromised patients. The choice should be based on the patient's medical history, the complexity of the procedure, and the patient's level of anxiety. Local anesthesia is often preferred, but in some cases, sedation may be required. In such instances, options like nitrous oxide (laughing gas), oral sedatives, or intravenous sedation can be considered. However, the patient's overall medical condition must be carefully assessed to ensure that these methods are safe for use.

   When administering anesthesia and sedation, it is crucial to be aware of potential drug interactions, especially in patients who are taking multiple medications for their medical conditions [21–23]. For example, certain sedatives may have interactions with drugs used to treat hypertension or diabetes. Prior consultation with the patient's primary healthcare provider or a pharmacist can help in identifying and managing these interactions. It's also essential to have a comprehensive understanding of the pharmacodynamics and pharmacokinetics of the anesthetics and sedatives used, to adjust dosages appropriately and monitor for any adverse reactions.

## 8.5 Intraoperative Management

1. Monitoring and Support

   Intraoperative management starts with vigilant monitoring of the patient's vital signs, including blood pressure, heart rate, oxygen saturation, and respiratory rate. Continuous monitoring is crucial for early detection of any adverse events. Additionally, the dental team should be prepared for potential emergencies. This includes having emergency protocols in place and ready access to emergency equipment, such as oxygen, defibrillators, and emergency drugs. Staff training in handling medical emergencies is also essential.

   Managing preexisting medical issues during the surgical procedure is a critical aspect of intraoperative care. For example, in patients with diabetes, maintaining stable blood glucose levels is important to prevent hyperglycemia or hypoglycemia [13]. In patients with cardiovascular diseases, maintaining hemodynamic stability is crucial [1]. Adjustments may need to be made in real-time based on the patient's response to the procedure and any changes in their condition.

2. Communication and Patient Comfort

   Effective communication with the patient throughout the procedure is vital. This involves explaining each step of the procedure to the patient, continually assessing their comfort level, and being responsive to their needs. Clear communication helps in reducing patient anxiety and ensures their cooperation during the procedure.

   Several techniques can be employed to reduce patient anxiety and discomfort during dental procedures. These can include:

   - Use of sedation: Depending on the patient's health status and anxiety level, various forms of sedation can be utilized.

- Distraction techniques: Providing distractions such as music, visual aids, or even simple conversation can help in easing patient anxiety.
- Pain management: Effective local anesthesia and postoperative pain management strategies are crucial for patient comfort.
- Gentle and reassuring chairside manner: The dental team's approach can significantly impact patient comfort and anxiety levels.

In certain situations, it may be necessary to refer the patient back to their primary care physician or a specialist. Such scenarios include the development of complications that are beyond the scope of dental management or when symptoms suggest a worsening of the patient's underlying medical condition. Effective communication with the patient's healthcare team is essential for coordinated care and optimal patient outcomes.

## 8.6 Postoperative Care and Complications

1. Postoperative Instructions

   Postoperative care should be customized according to the specific medical condition of the patient. For example, diabetic patients may require more frequent blood sugar monitoring after the procedure, while patients with cardiovascular disease might need closer observation for signs of bleeding or hemodynamic instability. The instructions may include guidelines on diet, activity level, oral hygiene practices, and signs of complications to watch for.

   Effective medication management is key in the postoperative period. This includes prescribing appropriate pain relievers that do not interfere with the patient's existing medication regimen, and in some cases, antibiotics to prevent infection. Adjustments to the patient's regular medications, such as anticoagulants, may also be necessary. Scheduling timely follow-up appointments is crucial to monitor the healing process and to address any concerns promptly.

2. Handling Complications

   Dental professionals should be vigilant in identifying and managing common postoperative complications such as infection, prolonged bleeding, or delayed healing. Knowledge of signs and symptoms that indicate complications is crucial for early intervention. For instance, excessive swelling, severe pain, or signs of infection at the extraction site should prompt immediate action.

## 8.7 Conclusion

The comprehensive examination of tooth extraction in medically compromised patients highlights the intricate balance between dental procedures and overall patient health. Special attention to patients with cardiovascular conditions, or other systemic health issues, is crucial due to the potential risks and complications associated with dental extractions. Understanding these medical complexities is not only essential for the safety and well-being of these individuals but also for the successful execution of dental procedures.

This discussion has emphasized the importance of a holistic approach to patient care, where dental practitioners must integrate their knowledge of oral health with a deep understanding of the patient's overall medical condition. The choice of anesthesia, the technique of extraction, and the management of postoperative care need to be meticulously tailored to each patient's unique health profile.

The insights provided in this chapter are invaluable for dental professionals who encounter medically compromised patients. They serve to enhance the quality of care and ensure that dental procedures, such as tooth extractions, are conducted with the utmost consideration for the patient's comprehensive health status. The knowledge shared here is vital for fostering a more informed and empathetic approach to dental care, ultimately contributing to better health outcomes for patients with complex medical backgrounds.

## References


1. Lu P, Gong Y, Chen Y, Cai W, Sheng J. Safety analysis of tooth extraction in elderly patients with cardiovascular diseases. Med Sci Monit. 2014;20:782–8. https://doi.org/10.12659/MSM.890131.
2. Inokoshi M, Kubota K, Yamaga E, Ueda K, Minakuchi S. Postoperative bleeding after dental extraction among elderly patients under anticoagulant therapy. Clin Oral Investig. 2021;25(4):2363–71. https://doi.org/10.1007/s00784-020-03559-z.
3. Moldovan MA, Filip LV, Ciurea M, et al. Bleeding and thromboembolic risk in patients under anticoagulant therapy receiving oral surgery: a systematic review. Med Pharm Rep. 2023;96(4):346–57. https://doi.org/10.15386/mpr-2519.
4. Dudek D, Marchionni S, Gabriele M, et al. Bleeding rate after tooth extraction in patients under oral anticoagulant therapy. J Craniofac Surg. 2016;27(5):1228–33. https://doi.org/10.1097/SCS.0000000000002713.
5. Yang S, Li Y, Liu C, Wu Y, Wan Z, Shen D. Pathogenesis and treatment of wound healing in patients with diabetes after tooth extraction. Front Endocrinol (Lausanne). 2022;13:949535. https://doi.org/10.3389/fendo.2022.949535.
6. Hong WW, Kim IH, Hong BM, Oak S, Mupparapu M. A patient presenting for dental extraction after completion of chemotherapy. Dent Clin N Am. 2023;67(4):667–70. https://doi.org/10.1016/j.cden.2023.05.020.
7. Akashi M, Kishimoto M, Kusumoto J, Yakushijin K, Matsuoka H, Komori T. Delayed socket healing after dental extraction in patients undergoing myelosuppressive chemotherapy for hematological malignancy: incidence and risk factors. J Oral Maxillofac Surg. 2018;76(10):2057–65. https://doi.org/10.1016/j.joms.2018.05.023.
8. Helenius-Hietala J, Aberg F, Meurman JH, Nordin A, Isoniemi H. Oral surgery in liver transplant candidates: a retrospective study on delayed bleeding and other complications. Oral Surg Oral Med Oral Pathol Oral Radiol. 2016;121(5):490–5. https://doi.org/10.1016/j.oooo.2016.01.025.
9. Eagle KA, Berger PB, Calkins H, et al. ACC/AHA guideline update for perioperative cardiovascular evaluation for noncardiac surgery---executive summary a report of the American College of Cardiology/American Heart Association Task Force on Practice Guidelines (Committee to Update the 1996 Guidelines on Perioperative Cardiovascular Evaluation for Noncardiac Surgery). Circulation. 2002;105(10):1257–67.
10. New York Heart Association. Diseases of the heart and blood vessels: nomenclature and criteria for diagnosis. 6th ed. Boston: Little, Brown; 1964.
11. Moster M, Bolliger D. Perioperative guidelines on antiplatelet and anticoagulant agents: 2022 update. Curr Anesthesiol Rep. 2022;12:286–96. https://doi.org/10.1007/s40140-021-00511-z.
12. Hirsh J, Fuster V, Ansell J, Halperin JL, American Heart Association, American College of Cardiology Foundation. American Heart Association/American College of Cardiology Foundation guide to warfarin therapy. Circulation. 2003;107(12):1692–711. https://doi.org/10.1161/01.CIR.0000063575.17904.4E.
13. Gazal G. Management of an emergency tooth extraction in diabetic patients on the dental chair. Saudi Dent J. 2020;32(1):1–6. https://doi.org/10.1016/j.sdentj.2019.07.004.
14. Moitra VK, Greenberg J, Arunajadai S, Sweitzer B. The relationship between glycosylated hemoglobin and perioperative glucose control in patients with diabetes. Can J Anaesth. 2010;57(4):322–9. https://doi.org/10.1007/s12630-010-9266-8.
15. Vegh D, Bencze B, Banyai D, et al. Preoperative HbA1c and blood glucose measurements in diabetes mellitus before oral surgery and implantology treatments. Int J Environ Res Public Health. 2023;20(6):4745. https://doi.org/10.3390/ijerph20064745.
16. Nakagawa Y, Shimada Y, Kawasaki Y, et al. Risk factors for post-tooth extraction complications in HIV-infected patients: a retrospective study. Jpn J Infect Dis. 2021;74(5):392–8. https://doi.org/10.7883/yoken.JJID.2019.273.
17. Figueiredo MA, Andrade NS, Blanco Carrion A, Medina JB, Gallottini M, Ortega KL. Bleeding during tooth extraction in patients with chronic kidney disease: a cross-sectional pilot study. Oral Dis. 2024;30:2617–24. https://doi.org/10.1111/odi.14709.
18. Sulejmanagic H, Sulejmanagic N, Prohic S, Secic S, Miseljic S. Dental treatment of patients with kidney diseases-review. Bosn J Basic Med Sci. 2005;5(1):52–6. https://doi.org/10.17305/bjbms.2005.3335.
19. Hupp WS. Dental management of patients with obstructive pulmonary diseases. Dent Clin N Am. 2006;50(4):513–27, vi. https://doi.org/10.1016/j.cden.2006.06.005.
20. Ruggiero SL, Dodson TB, Aghaloo T, Carlson ER, Ward BB, Kademani D. American Association of Oral and Maxillofacial Surgeons' position paper on medication-related osteonecrosis of the Jaws-2022 update. J Oral Maxillofac Surg. 2022;80(5):920–43. https://doi.org/10.1016/j.joms.2022.02.008.
21. Cullen BF, Miller MG. Drug interactions and anesthesia: a review. Anesth Analg. 1979;58(5):413–23. https://doi.org/10.1213/00000539-197909000-00014.
22. Milaszkiewicz RM. Diabetes mellitus and anesthesia: what is the problem? Int Anesthesiol Clin. 1997;35(4):35–62. https://doi.org/10.1097/00004311-199703540-00004.
23. McAnulty GR, Robertshaw HJ, Hall GM. Anaesthetic management of patients with diabetes mellitus. Br J Anaesth. 2000;85(1):80–90. https://doi.org/10.1093/bja/85.1.80.

# Extraction for the Child

# 9

## Contents



## 9.1 Introduction

Children are a unique demographic when it comes to dental care. Their physiological, psychological, and developmental needs differ significantly from adults, necessitating a tailored approach to their oral health [1]. This is particularly true in the context of tooth extraction, a procedure that, while common, requires careful consideration and a specialized approach when performed on children.

Primary teeth, often referred to as "baby teeth," play a crucial role in a child's development. They are not merely placeholders for permanent teeth but are vital for chewing, speaking, and maintaining space for the eventual eruption of permanent teeth. The extraction of these teeth, therefore, is not a decision to be taken lightly. It involves a comprehensive understanding of the indications and contraindications specific to pediatric patients.

Indications for the extraction of primary teeth in children may include severe decay, infection, orthodontic reasons, or trauma. However, each case must be evaluated on its own merits, considering the child's overall health, the condition of the tooth, and the potential impact on the child's oral and general development. On the other hand,


S.-G. Kim et al., *Advanced Strategies for Tooth Extraction in Dentistry*,
https://doi.org/10.1007/978-981-97-6532-4_9

contraindications might include certain medical conditions, acute infections, or the lack of a clear benefit to the child's oral health.

Before proceeding with an extraction, it is imperative to consider various factors. These include the child's age, the stage of dental development, the presence of underlying medical conditions, and the potential for psychological impact. The child's emotional and cognitive maturity must be assessed to determine the best approach for managing their anxiety and ensuring their comfort throughout the procedure.

The extraction of a primary tooth is not the end of the treatment but rather a part of a broader, ongoing dental care plan. Post-extraction considerations include monitoring the healing process, managing any discomfort, and planning for the future eruption of permanent teeth. Space maintainers may be necessary to prevent space loss and subsequent misalignment of the permanent teeth.

Moreover, the role of the dentist extends beyond the technical execution of the extraction. It involves educating and communicating effectively with both the child and their guardians. Guardians must be fully informed about the reasons for the extraction, the procedure itself, and the postoperative care required. Children, too, require an explanation appropriate to their level of understanding, ensuring they are reassured and cooperative.

In summary, tooth extraction in children is a procedure that demands a specialized approach, considering the unique implications on their development and the necessity for a supportive, informative environment. As dental professionals, our goal is to ensure the health and well-being of the child, guiding them and their guardians through the process with care, expertise, and empathy. This chapter will delve into the intricacies of pediatric tooth extraction, providing a comprehensive guide for those entrusted with the delicate task of caring for a child's oral health.

## 9.2 Indication of Extracting a Primary Tooth

The decision to extract a primary tooth in a child is one that must be approached with careful consideration. Several clinical scenarios warrant this intervention, each with its implications and requirements. This section will outline the primary indications for primary tooth extraction, providing a framework for understanding when and why these procedures are necessary.

1. Severe Decay of the Crown

   One of the most common reasons for extracting a primary tooth is when the crown is severely decayed. In such cases, the decay may be so extensive that restoration is impractical or impossible. If left untreated, this can lead to pain, infection, and potential damage to the underlying permanent tooth. Early intervention is crucial to prevent more severe complications and ensure the child's overall oral health.
2. Lesions on the Root

   Lesions on the root of a primary tooth can pose a significant risk to the developing permanent tooth beneath. These lesions may be cystic or tumorous in nature and can cause damage to the underlying structures if not addressed promptly. Extraction is often necessary to remove the lesion and prevent any detrimental effects on the permanent tooth's eruption and health.
3. Odontogenic Abscesses

   Primary teeth that are the cause of odontogenic abscesses require extraction to resolve the infection and prevent its spread. An abscess can be extremely painful and may lead to more significant health issues if the infection reaches other areas of the body. Prompt extraction, coupled with appropriate antibiotic treatment, is essential to manage these cases effectively.
4. Fractured Root Due to Trauma

   Traumatic injuries can result in fractured roots of primary teeth. In such instances, extraction is often the only viable option to alleviate pain and prevent potential infection.

It's also important to consider the psychological impact of trauma on the child and provide appropriate support and reassurance throughout the treatment process.

5. Hindrance to Normal Eruption of Permanent Teeth

   In some cases, a primary tooth may be malpositioned or retained longer than usual, obstructing the normal eruption of a permanent tooth. Timely extraction of the primary tooth can provide the necessary space for the permanent tooth to erupt correctly, preventing future alignment issues and more complex orthodontic treatments.

6. Problematic Neonatal Teeth

   Neonatal teeth, those that are present at birth or emerge within the first month of life, can sometimes pose problems during nursing and may be at risk of aspiration. If these teeth are loose, cause irritation to the infant or mother during nursing, or pose other health risks, extraction might be necessary to alleviate these issues and prevent more severe complications.

The extraction of primary teeth in children may be indicated in various situations, each requiring a thoughtful, case-by-case assessment. Understanding the specific reasons and the broader implications of these extractions is crucial for dental professionals. It enables them to provide the most appropriate care, ensuring the child's immediate comfort and long-term oral health. As we move forward, it is important to remember that each child is unique, and the approach to their dental care should be just as personalized, considering all aspects of their health and well-being.

## 9.3 Contraindication of Extracting a Primary Tooth

While the extraction of primary teeth can be necessary for various reasons, there are specific situations where the procedure may need to be postponed, modified, or approached with extreme caution. Understanding these contraindications is crucial to ensure the safety and well-being of the child. This section will discuss the primary contraindications for primary tooth extraction and the considerations that must be taken into account.

1. Systemic Diseases Such as Congenital Heart Disease

   Children with systemic conditions, particularly those affecting the heart, pose a unique challenge when it comes to dental extractions. Conditions like congenital heart disease can increase the risk of complications during and after the procedure. For these children, it is essential to consult with a specialist in the field before proceeding. The specialist can provide guidance on the safest approach, including the need for prophylactic antibiotics or specific timing for the procedure to minimize risks. Collaboration between the dentist and the child's medical team is crucial to ensure a comprehensive approach to the child's health.

2. Rapid Progression of Infections

   Infections in children, particularly those around the oral cavity, can progress rapidly. If a child is already showing of fever, swelling, or cellulitis prior to the tooth extraction, it is imperative to reevaluate the situation promptly. In some cases, the child may require antibiotic treatment prior to extraction to manage the infection effectively. It is also important to monitor the child closely for any signs of systemic involvement, such as fever or malaise, which may indicate a more serious condition requiring immediate medical attention.

3. Considerations for Post-Extraction Care

   Even in the absence of systemic diseases or immediate complications, certain conditions may contraindicate extraction or necessitate special care. Children with bleeding disorders, immune deficiencies, or those undergoing chemotherapy or radiation therapy require careful planning and coordination with their medical team. In these cases, the risks of extraction must be weighed against the potential benefits, and all possible precautions should be taken to ensure the child's safety.

4. Communication and Informed Consent

   Finally, it is vital to maintain open and clear communication with the child's guardians and, when appropriate, the child themselves. They should be fully informed of the potential risks and benefits of the procedure, any contraindications, and the recommended course of action. Informed consent is a critical component of ethical and effective pediatric dental care.

In conclusion, while the extraction of primary teeth is a common procedure, it is not without its risks and contraindications. Dental professionals must be vigilant in recognizing these contraindications and proceed with caution, particularly in children with systemic diseases or those showing signs of infection. Collaboration with medical specialists, careful monitoring, and clear communication with the child and their guardians are key to ensuring a safe and successful outcome. As we continue to explore the nuances of pediatric dental care, it is clear that a thorough understanding of both the indications and contraindications for procedures like tooth extraction is essential.

## 9.4 Pre-Extraction Considerations in a Child

The decision to extract a tooth in a child is not just a dental procedure, but a significant event in the child's life. It is imperative that this process is approached with care, understanding, and thorough preparation. This chapter focuses on the essential considerations that must be taken before extracting a primary tooth, emphasizing the importance of communication, diagnostic preparations, and the coordination of care.

1. Communication with Guardians and Child

   Effective communication is the cornerstone of pediatric dentistry. Guardians must be provided with detailed information about why the extraction is necessary, what it entails, potential pain during the procedure, and strategies for behavior management. It is important to address any questions or concerns they may have openly and honestly. This not only helps in obtaining informed consent but also in building trust and ensuring cooperation throughout the process. Similarly, explaining the procedure to the child is equally important. This should be done using simple, nonthreatening terms. Children should understand why the extraction is necessary, what to expect during the procedure, and that they might feel some discomfort during anesthesia. It is also vital to be honest about any pain they may experience while ensuring them that it will be managed and is only temporary. Post-extraction precautions, such as not inserting fingers into the mouth and consuming only cold food for the day, should also be explained in a child-friendly manner.
2. Radiographic Assessment

   Before proceeding with an extraction, a thorough radiographic evaluation is essential. Imaging, typically a panoramic and standard view, helps assess several crucial factors:

   (a) Degree of root resorption: Understanding how much of the primary tooth's root remains is vital for planning the extraction and anticipating the ease or complexity of the procedure.
   (b) Presence of apical lesions: Identifying any lesions at the root's tip can indicate underlying pathology that might affect the procedure or necessitate additional treatment.
   (c) Position of permanent teeth: Knowing the location and developmental stage of the underlying permanent teeth helps in predicting the timing of their eruption and the need for any orthodontic intervention post-extraction.

If a permanent tooth is not expected to erupt immediately after the extraction of a primary tooth, planning for a space maintainer is essential. This device helps prevent the shifting of adjacent teeth into the gap, ensuring the proper spacing for the eventual eruption of the permanent tooth. The space maintainer should be prepared in advance and fitted immediately after the extraction to be most effective. Ectopic eruption, particularly of the maxillary canines, is a concern in pediatric dentistry. Occurring in about 3–9% of cases, these teeth often emerge palatally and can disrupt the

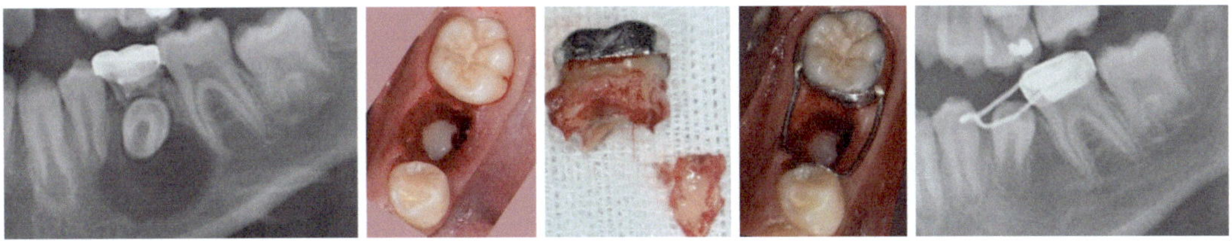

**Fig. 9.1** Extraction of primary molar and space maintaining (by Courtesy of prof. Lee EK)

alignment of the dental arch [2]. In such cases, early consultation with an orthodontist and a pediatric dentist is crucial. These specialists can help determine the best timing for the extraction of the ectopic tooth and any other interventions that may be necessary to guide the proper eruption and alignment of the teeth.

Pre-extraction considerations are crucial in ensuring the success and smoothness of the procedure. By addressing these aspects—communication, diagnostic preparations, and planning for the aftermath—dental professionals can provide a more comprehensive and considerate care for their pediatric patients. As we delve deeper into the nuances of pediatric tooth extraction, it becomes increasingly clear that the procedure is as much about the technical aspects of dentistry as it is about understanding and catering to the unique needs of children (Fig. 9.1).

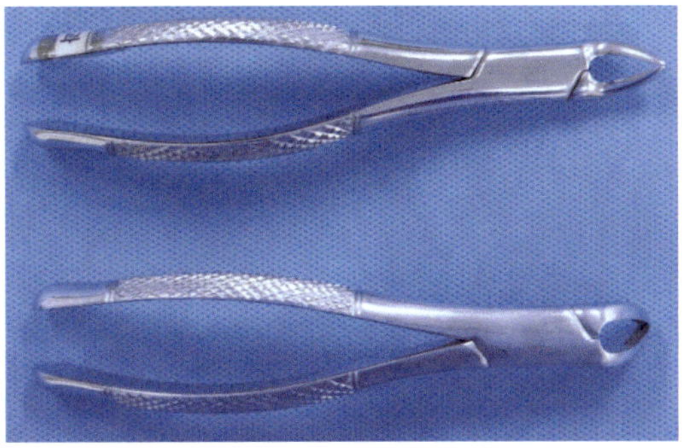

**Fig. 9.2** Pediatric forceps for primary teeth extraction. #150S (above) and #151S (below)

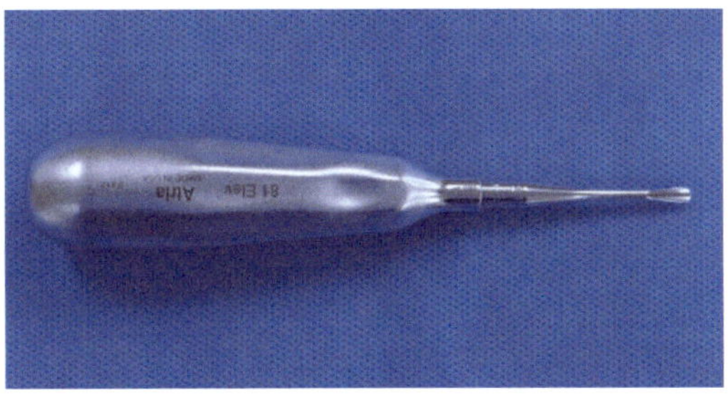

**Fig. 9.3** Pediatric elevator for primary teeth extraction

## 9.5 Extraction Method for Deciduous Tooth

### 9.5.1 Instrument for the Primary Teeth Extraction

1. Pediatric Forceps

   These are smaller and more delicate than adult forceps to accommodate the smaller size and more fragile nature of primary teeth (Fig. 9.2). They are designed to fit the smaller mouth of a child and to grasp the smaller crowns of deciduous teeth effectively without imposing undue pressure on adjacent teeth or soft tissues. Different types are available for different teeth (anterior vs. posterior).

   (a) #150S (upper universal forceps for children): A smaller version of the standard #150 forceps used for adults, designed for extracting upper primary teeth. The "S" denotes the smaller size suitable for children.
   (b) #151S (lower universal forceps for children): A smaller version of the #151 forceps used for lower teeth in adults, adapted for extracting lower primary teeth in children.
   (c) #150AS and #151AS: These are similar to the #150S and #151S but with a more pronounced beak angle, designed to accommodate the anatomy of primary molars.

2. Elevators

   Pediatric elevators are also smaller and used to loosen the tooth from the periodontal ligament before extraction (Fig. 9.3). They

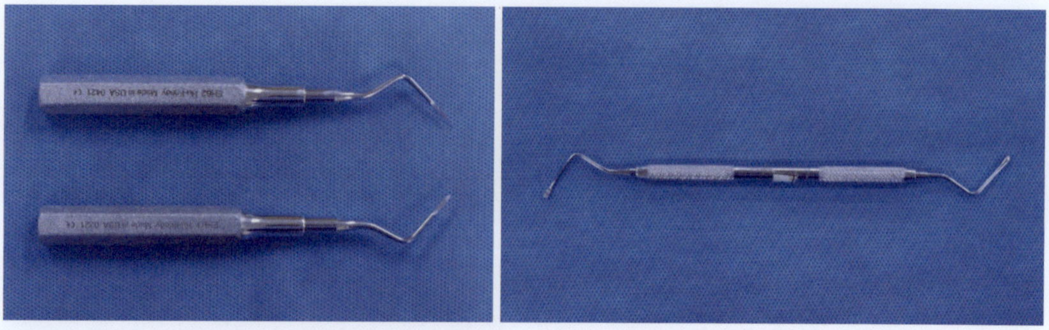

**Fig. 9.4** Root picks (left) and small alveolar curette (right)

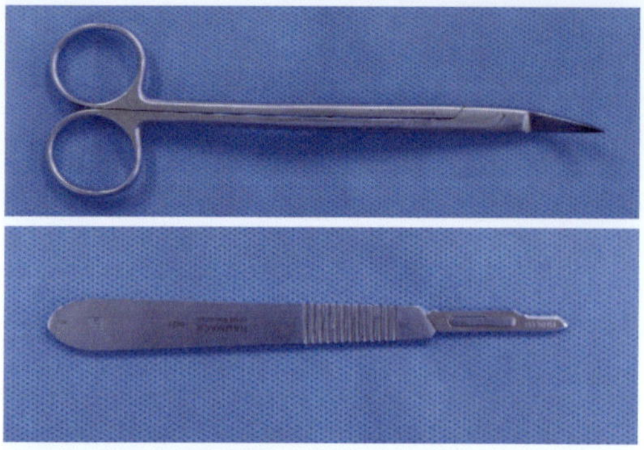

**Fig. 9.5** Dental scissor (above) and scalpel (below)

help to expand the socket and separate the tooth from its ligament with minimal damage to surrounding tissues. Care is taken to use them gently to avoid damaging the developing permanent teeth underneath. Although not forceps, Warwick James elevators are often used in pediatric dentistry to loosen primary teeth before extraction. They come in straight, left, and right versions to adapt to different teeth and positions.

3. Root Picks or Small Curettes

   These are used if the deciduous tooth is broken or if roots remain in the socket after the crown has been removed (Fig. 9.4). They are designed to carefully remove the remaining pieces without disturbing the underlying permanent tooth.

4. Dental Scissors and Scalpels

   These might be used to make a small incision in the gum tissue to access a tooth that has not erupted fully or to remove soft tissue overgrowths (Fig. 9.5).

5. Syringes and Needles

   Smaller gauge needles are used to administer local anesthesia in children to make the procedure as comfortable as possible (Fig. 9.6).

6. Mouth Props

   These are used to help keep a child's mouth open during the procedure. They are smaller and designed to fit comfortably in a child's mouth (Fig. 9.7).

7. Bite Blocks

   Similar to mouth props, bite blocks help keep the mouth open and reduce fatigue in the jaw muscles during longer procedures (Fig. 9.8).

8. Suction Devices

   Smaller suction tips are used to clear saliva, blood, and debris from the child's mouth without causing discomfort or trauma (Fig. 9.9).

9. Rubber Dams

   These might be used to isolate the tooth being worked on, to prevent aspiration of the tooth or other materials, and to provide a clean working area (Fig. 9.10).

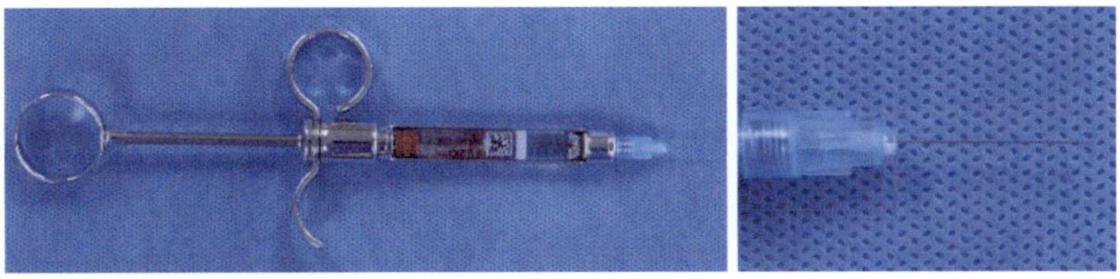

**Fig. 9.6** Syringe and needle

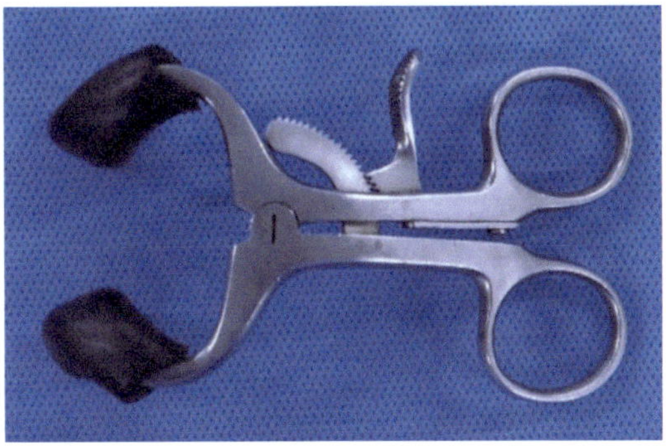

**Fig. 9.7** Mouth prop

The instruments are used with a gentle touch to avoid damaging the delicate tissues in a child's mouth and the developing permanent teeth beneath the primary teeth. Some pediatric dental instruments might be designed or decorated in a way that appears more child-friendly, helping to reduce anxiety and make the experience less intimidating. Like all dental instruments, those used for children must be properly sterilized to prevent infection.

When extracting deciduous teeth, the primary goal is to perform the procedure effectively while causing minimal discomfort and avoiding any damage to the developing permanent teeth. Therefore, the choice and use of instruments are carried out with precision and care, tailored to the unique needs of pediatric patients (Fig. 9.11).

### 9.5.2 Extraction of Primary Incisor

1. Root resorption in maxillary primary incisors typically begins at the apical portion on the palatal side and proceeds vertically, often leaving only the crown, which then becomes loose. In cases of moderate or greater mobility, forceps can be used to easily extract the tooth. Generally, it is recommended to extract these teeth after confirming the position of the permanent tooth. If there is little to no root resorption in a maxillary primary incisor, it is advisable to perform a rotational movement around the tooth axis to luxate the tooth before extracting it buccally. In cases where the root is moderately resorbed, with the apex remaining thin and adhered to the buccal alveolar bone, it is beneficial to separate the root from the buccal wall and extract it in the palatal direction. When more than two-thirds of the root is resorbed, rotating around the tooth axis to luxate the tooth and then extracting it in the palatal direction is a method that allows extraction without root fracture.
2. In the case of mandibular primary incisors, as the roots are thinner and longer compared to maxillary incisors, there is a higher incidence of root fracture, so care must be taken during extraction. Particularly, since lingual eruption occurs in about 18.4% of cases, extraction should be performed immediately if lingual eruption is confirmed, even in the absence of mobility [3].

### 9.5.3 Extraction of Primary Molar

1. Maxillary primary molars have three roots, while mandibular primary molars have two. Permanent teeth typically begin to erupt between these roots. The onset of resorption of the roots of primary molars coincides with

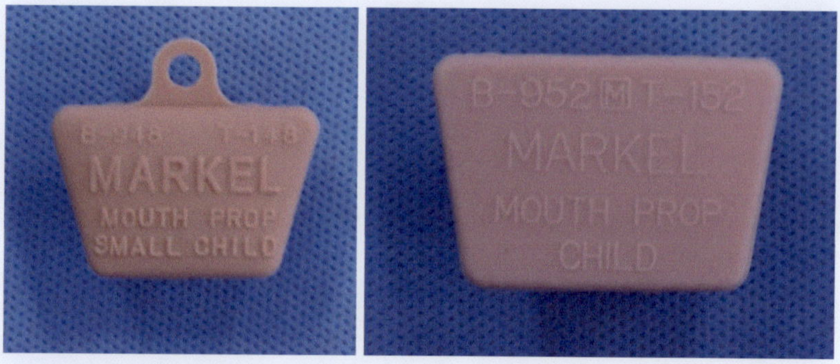


**Fig. 9.8** Small bite block for the child

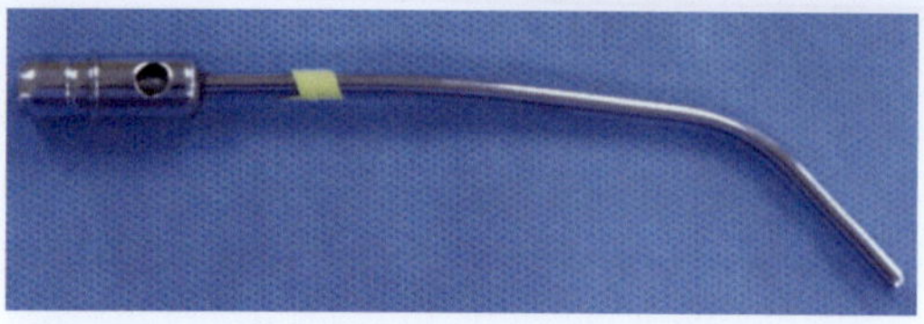

**Fig. 9.9** Small suction tip (9 French)

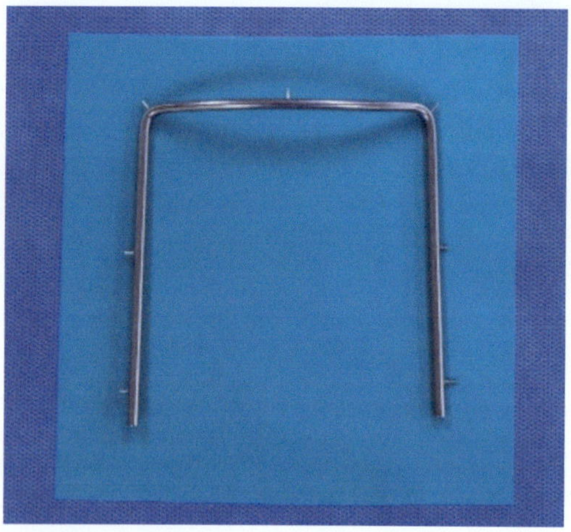

**Fig. 9.10** Rubber dam

the eruption of permanent teeth, and the degree of root resorption significantly influences the difficulty of extraction.

2. In cases where there is little to no root resorption, it is advisable to use a bur to separate the roots and then extract them one by one. However, care must be taken as this method may cause damage to the emerging permanent teeth. Therefore, it is recommended to perform the extraction when some mobility of the primary molar is observed following root resorption.
3. If root fracture occurs during extraction, it is better not to forcefully remove it and leave it as it is (Fig. 9.12). In most cases, the remaining root fragments will either be resorbed as the permanent tooth erupts or will be pushed up and can be easily removed later.

### 9.5.4 Extraction of Fused Tooth

Fusion refers to a developmental anomaly where two teeth are united. It is often confused with gemination (Fig. 9.13). Typically, a fused tooth is characterized by joined enamel and/or dentin and may have two roots or a single root with two canals. In contrast, a geminated tooth usually presents with two crowns and a single root. Fused teeth occur in about 0.1–1.6% of cases, predominantly in the anterior region [4]. The decision to extract a fused tooth should take into account the presence and eruption status of the permanent teeth.

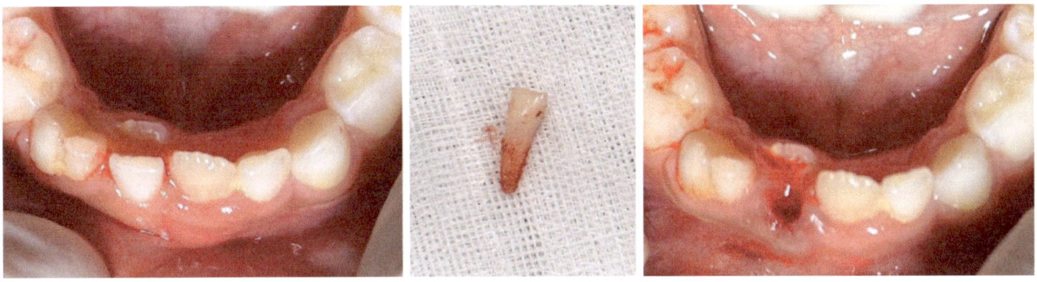

**Fig. 9.11** Extraction of mandibular primary incisor (by Courtesy of Dr. Jeong CS)

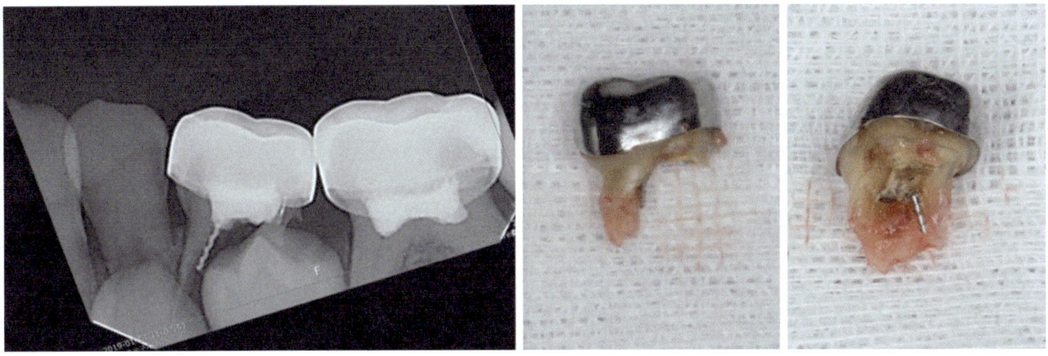

**Fig. 9.12** Extraction of mandibular primary molar (by Courtesy of prof. Lee EK)

**Fig. 9.13** Extraction of fused tooth (by Courtesy of prof. Lee EK)

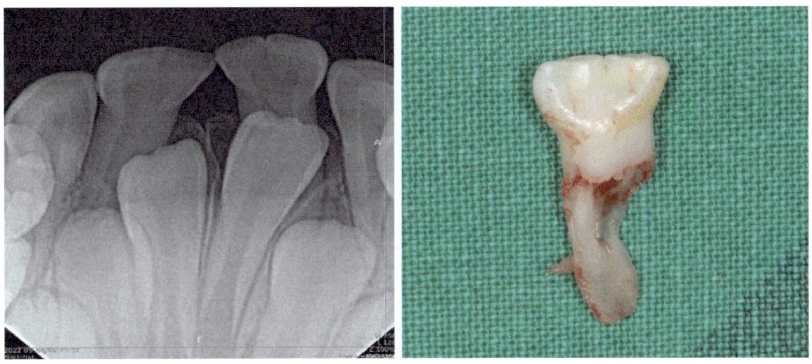

## 9.6 Post-Extraction Care in a Child

The period following the extraction of a primary tooth is critical for a child's recovery and long-term oral health. Children's post-extraction care differs from adults due to their unique physiological and developmental needs. This chapter focuses on the essential post-extraction care strategies to ensure proper healing and comfort for the child.

1. Care of the Extraction Site

   After the extraction, it is crucial to manage the socket with care. Excessive curettage should be avoided to prevent damage to the underlying permanent teeth and to reduce the risk of excessive bleeding. Only inflammatory tissue should be gently removed. The goal is to promote natural healing, minimize discomfort, and prevent damage to the developing permanent tooth. Guardians should be instructed on how to monitor the site for signs of infection or unusual bleeding and to contact their dentist if they have any concerns.

2. Managing Food Intake

   The effects of anesthesia can linger, causing numbness in the mouth, which increases the risk of the child biting their tongue or lips. To prevent this, food intake should be limited until the anesthesia wears off completely. Guardians should closely monitor the child during this period and provide appropriate care to ensure the child does not injure themselves unknowingly.

3. Installation of Space Maintainers

   If there is a need to maintain the space until the eruption of the permanent teeth, a space maintainer should be installed. This device is crucial in preventing the neighboring teeth from drifting into the gap left by the extracted tooth, which could lead to alignment issues or impaction of the permanent tooth. The timing of the installation and the type of space maintainer will vary depending on the child's age, which tooth was extracted, and the expected time for the eruption of the permanent tooth.

4. Dietary Recommendations

   On the day of the extraction, it is advisable for the child to consume cold, nonacidic, and soft foods. These types of foods are less likely to irritate the extraction site and are easier to eat when the mouth is numb. Recommended options include ice cream, yogurt, milkshakes, mashed potatoes, oatmeal, and scrambled eggs. These foods not only comfort the child but also provide the necessary nutrition for recovery. A normal diet can usually be resumed the day after extraction, once hemostasis is confirmed and the child feels comfortable.

Effective post-extraction care is crucial in ensuring a smooth and comfortable recovery for the child. By paying careful attention to the extraction site, managing food intake, installing space maintainers when necessary, and providing appropriate dietary recommendations, guardians and dental professionals can help the child recover quickly and with minimal discomfort. Communication about these care strategies is essential, and guardians should feel well-informed and equipped to support their child through the recovery process. As dental professionals, our role extends beyond the procedure itself to providing comprehensive care that addresses the child's immediate and long-term oral health needs.

## 9.7 Conclusion

This chapter describes the indications, contraindications, pre-extraction considerations, and post-extraction care for primary tooth extraction. It provides detailed explanations of the points to be cautious about when extracting primary teeth and primary molars in children.

## References

1. Cha IH, Yu JH, Lee JH, et al. Textbook of oral and maxillofacial surgery. 4th ed. Koonja Publisher; 2023. p. 108–10.
2. Habib A, Athanasiou AE, Makrygiannakis MA, et al. Do the various interceptive treatment modalities improve the position of palatally displaced permanent canines? A meta-analysis. Eur J Orthod. 2023;45:370–81. https://doi.org/10.1093/ejo/cjac076.
3. Aminabadi NA, Farahani RM, Pouralibaba AS. Lingual eruption of mandibular permanent incisors: a space correlated phenomenon? J Contemp Dent Pract. 2009;10(1):25–32. https://thejcdp.com/doi/JCDP/pdf/10.5005/jcdp-10-1-25
4. Sekerci AE, Sisman Y, Ekizer A, et al. Prevalence of double (fused/geminated) primary teeth in Turkey - a study. Pak Oral Dent J. 2011;31(1):1–7. https://www.proquest.com/docview/1038334294?pq-origsite=gscholar&fromopenview=true&sourcetype=Scholarly%20Journals

# Intentional Replantation and Transplantation

# 10

## Contents



## 10.1 Introduction

Autotransplantation, a technique in the field of dental surgery, involves the strategic relocation of teeth within the same individual's mouth [1]. It serves as a promising option for addressing various dental issues, including tooth loss or misalignment. This procedure can be broadly categorized into three distinct types based on the destination of the extracted tooth. The first category is transplantation. Here, an extracted tooth is moved and implanted into a different location within the mouth. This technique is often employed when there is a need to fill a gap left by a missing tooth, utilizing another tooth that may be extraneous or improperly positioned.

The second type, known as intentional replantation, involves the extraction of a tooth followed by necessary treatments and its subsequent reinsertion into its original socket. This procedure is typically considered when the tooth in question is viable for restoration but is afflicted with conditions, such as root canal issues, that are unresolvable while it remains in situ. Lastly, surgical repositioning refers to the minor adjustment or uprighting of a tooth within its existing socket. This method is generally applied to correct misaligned teeth that do not require full extraction and transplantation but rather a slight positional correction within the same dental socket [2].

The success of autotransplantation procedures heavily relies on meticulous presurgical case selection. One of the critical factors in choosing a suitable donor tooth is its mesiodistal distance, which must match precisely with that of the recipient site to ensure a proper fit and optimal healing conditions. The donor tooth's shape, size, and root development stage are also vital considerations, as these factors significantly influence the transplant's viability and long-term success.

Furthermore, it is essential to recognize that, like all surgical interventions, autotransplantation carries potential risks and complications. These may include tooth loss, failure of the tooth


S.-G. Kim et al., *Advanced Strategies for Tooth Extraction in Dentistry*,
https://doi.org/10.1007/978-981-97-6532-4_10

to integrate into its new position, and various postoperative issues like infection or resorption. Therefore, a thorough patient consultation is crucial. This includes a comprehensive discussion about the potential risks, expected outcomes, and the necessity of postoperative care. Ensuring that patients are fully informed and providing their informed consent is not just a legal obligation but a fundamental ethical practice, ensuring that they are active, informed participants in their care plan. Autotransplantation, encompassing transplantation, intentional replantation, and surgical repositioning, offers a versatile set of options for addressing various dental conditions. With careful planning, precise execution, and thorough patient consultation, these procedures can significantly improve dental health and patient well-being. As we delve deeper into this chapter, we will explore the detailed methodologies, case studies, and innovations that make autotransplantation a valuable tool in modern dentistry.

## 10.2 Intentional Replantation

1. Indication

   Intentional replantation is a specialized dental procedure employed under specific circumstances where traditional approaches, such as conventional root canal treatment, are either not possible or have failed to alleviate pain. This section delineates the scenarios where intentional replantation is considered a viable option.

   (a) Instrument fracture during root canal treatment:

   One of the primary indications for intentional replantation is the occurrence of instrument fracture during root canal therapy. At times, the instruments used to clean or shape the canal may break and become lodged within the canal. If these fractured pieces cannot be retrieved and are accompanied by persistent pain, intentional replantation offers an alternative solution. In this process, the tooth is extracted, the fractured instrument is removed, and necessary treatments are administered before the tooth is reinserted into its original socket.

   (b) Re-treatment challenges due to posts or pins:

   In certain cases, a tooth that has previously undergone root canal treatment may require re-treatment due to persistent issues. However, the presence of posts or pins, which are used to rebuild and strengthen the tooth structure, can make access to the root canal complicated or impossible. If such a situation is accompanied by ongoing pain, intentional replantation can be considered to effectively address the issue without the constraints posed by the posts or pins.

   (c) Overextension of root canal filling material:

   Sometimes, the material used to fill the root canal after cleaning may extend beyond the root apex. This overextension can lead to irritation and pain in the surrounding tissues. If the pain persists and conventional treatment methods are ineffective, intentional replantation can be utilized. The tooth is extracted, the overextended filling material is corrected, and any necessary treatments are conducted before the tooth is reinserted.

   (d) Canal stenosis with complications:

   Canal stenosis, a condition characterized by the narrowing or blockage of the root canal, can make root canal treatment challenging or unfeasible. If this condition is accompanied by a periapical lesion or ongoing pain, it becomes essential to find an alternative solution. Intentional replantation allows for the direct access and treatment of the problem area. After extraction, the necessary procedures are carried out to address the stenosis, periapical lesion, or pain before the tooth is replanted.

   In each of these scenarios, the goal of intentional replantation is to preserve the natural tooth and maintain its function in the oral cavity. This procedure is not without its risks and requires careful consideration and planning. The potential for complications, such as resorption or ankylosis, underscores the importance of a thorough diagnostic process, precise surgical technique, and comprehensive postoperative care. It is imperative that patients are well-informed about the procedure, its benefits, risks, and the necessary aftercare to ensure the best possible outcome. As we proceed, we will further explore the methodology, procedural nuances, and care considerations integral to the successful application of intentional replantation in clinical practice.

2. Surgical Procedure

The surgical procedure for intentional replantation is a meticulous process designed to preserve the natural tooth while addressing underlying dental issues. This section outlines the step-by-step approach undertaken during this intricate surgery (Fig. 10.1).

(a) Presurgical preparation:

Prior to surgery, it is vital to establish a healthy environment around the surgical area. This includes caries control and periodontal treatment to ensure that the surrounding teeth and gums are in optimal condition and to minimize the risk of postoperative infection.

(b) Disinfection of the surgical site:

Once the area is prepared, the next step involves thoroughly disinfecting the surgical site. Iodine or chlorhexidine can be used to sterilize the area, significantly reducing the risk of infection during and after the procedure.

(c) Local anesthesia:

To ensure patient comfort and to facilitate a smooth surgical procedure, local anesthesia is administered to the area surrounding the tooth to be replanted. This helps in pain-free extraction and manipulation of the tooth.

(d) Gingival flap elevation:

A gingival flap is carefully elevated to expose the root of the tooth. This is a critical step as it provides access to the tooth and the surrounding bone, allowing for precise extraction and treatment.

(e) Tooth extraction:

The tooth intended for replantation is carefully extracted to preserve as much of the root structure as possible. Once extracted, the tooth is immediately placed

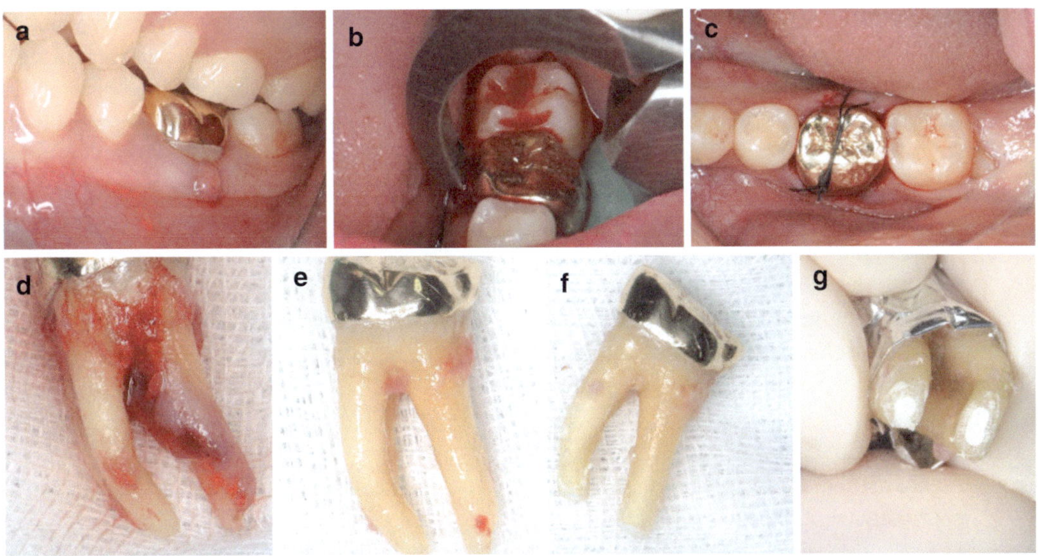

**Fig. 10.1** Surgical procedure. (**a**) Preoperative photo, (**b**) intraoperative photo of extraction, (**c**) fixation of the donor tooth using sutures after transplantation, (**d**) extracted tooth, (**e**) after root planning, (**f**) after apicoectomy, (**g**) after retrograde filling using MTA (by Courtesy of prof. Son SA)

in a saline solution to maintain its viability.

(f) Socket curettage:

With the tooth removed, the socket is gently curetted to remove any inflammatory tissue and foreign material. This step is crucial for preventing postoperative complications and ensuring a clean environment for the replanted tooth.

(g) Root examination and planning:

The extracted root is then examined for any attached lesions. These are removed, and root planning is performed to smoothen the root surface and facilitate better reintegration into the socket.

(h) Apicoectomy:

Holding the extracted tooth carefully, an apicoectomy is performed using a diamond bur. This involves the removal of the root tip and any surrounding infected tissue, a critical step for preventing future complications.

(i) Retrograde filling:

A retrograde filling using mineral trioxide aggregate (MTA) is then conducted. This material is placed at the end of the root canal to seal it off from the surrounding tissue, preventing leakage and infection.

(j) Socket disinfection and replantation:

Before replanting the tooth, the extraction socket is disinfected again with saline solution. The tooth is then gently reimplanted into the alveolus, ensuring it fits snugly and correctly.

(k) Tooth stabilization:

Once the tooth is in place, it is stabilized with suturing. Care is taken to eliminate any occlusal interference that might disrupt the healing process or cause discomfort.

(l) Postoperative care:

The stitches are typically removed approximately 2 weeks after the surgery. During the first week post-surgery, patients are advised to maintain a liquid diet and cleanse the area using chlorhexidine to promote healing and prevent infection.

The success of this procedure heavily depends on meticulous execution and careful postoperative care. Each step, from presurgical preparation to postoperative maintenance, plays a crucial role in ensuring the best possible outcome for the patient (Fig. 10.2). As we continue, we will delve into the critical postoperative considerations and long-term care necessary for the sustained success of intentional replantation.

3. Prognosis and Considerations

The prognosis for intentionally replanted teeth is contingent upon a multitude of factors, ranging from the immediate postoperative period through to the long-term maintenance of the tooth. Understanding these factors is crucial for anticipating outcomes and managing expectations. This section discusses the critical aspects influencing the prognosis and the necessary considerations for intentional replantation.

(a) Periodic clinical and radiographic examinations:

After the replantation procedure, it is imperative to conduct periodic clinical and radiographic examinations. These assessments aim to monitor the reattachment of the gingiva and periodontal ligament, the presence of progressive inflammation, and the development of ankylosis. These examinations provide valuable insights into the healing process and the overall success of the procedure [3].

(b) Vitality of the periodontal ligament:

The success rate of the replanted tooth is significantly higher if the periodontal ligament remains vital [4]. The periodontal ligament plays a crucial role in the tooth's reintegration into the alveolar bone. Damage to this ligament can lead to ankylosis (fusion of the tooth to the bone) or inflammatory root resorption, both of which are associated with a poor prognosis.

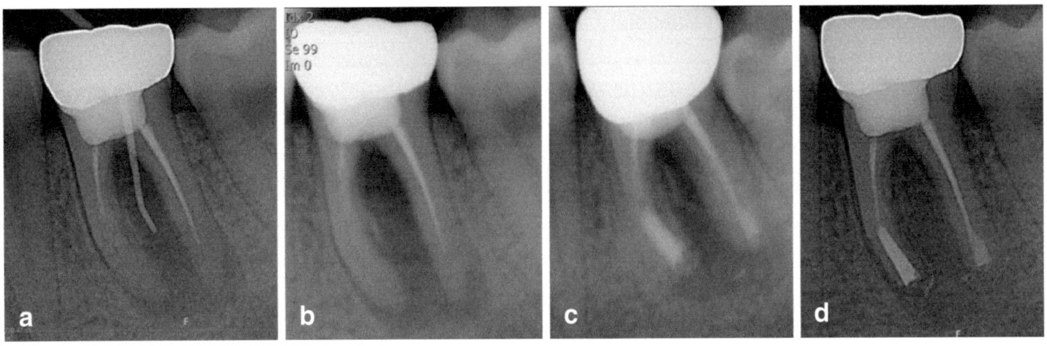


**Fig. 10.2** X-ray view before and after intentional replantation. (**a**) Gutta percha tracing on first visit, (**b**) preoperative X-ray, (**c**) immediate after replantation, (**d**) 6 months after replantation (by Courtesy of prof. Son SA)

(c) Ankylosis and functionality:

While ankylosis is generally considered an unfavorable outcome, there are instances where an ankylosed tooth maintains robust fixation and functionality for years. However, the long-term viability of such teeth remains uncertain, and they require ongoing monitoring.

(d) Root shape and extraction difficulty:

The shape of the root significantly influences the difficulty of extraction and, consequently, the prognosis. Teeth with complex root structures, like impacted teeth, typically have a poorer prognosis compared to those with simpler structures. This is due to the challenges associated with extracting such teeth without damaging the periodontal ligament and the matching of the root shape with the donor site.

(e) Tooth development stage:

The developmental stage of the tooth at the time of replantation also affects the prognosis. Generally, the replantation of a mature tooth has a less-favorable prognosis compared to a developing tooth. Developing teeth often have a more robust healing capacity and potential for successful reintegration.

(f) Method of fixation:

The method and duration of tooth fixation post-replantation are crucial. Teeth that are rigidly splinted for an extended period typically exhibit a higher incidence of root resorption, which can undermine the long-term success of the procedure [4]. Finding the right balance in fixation to allow for healing while minimizing adverse outcomes is key.

(g) Impact of root canal therapy:

The effect of root canal therapy on the prognosis of replanted teeth remains a subject of debate and uncertainty [5, 6]. While root canal therapy is a common component of the replantation process, its long-term impact on the success of the procedure requires further investigation.

The prognosis of intentionally replanted teeth is influenced by a complex interplay of factors. Thorough preoperative planning, precise surgical technique, and diligent postoperative care are fundamental to optimizing outcomes. Regular follow-ups and monitoring are essential for detecting and addressing potential complications early. By understanding and considering these various factors, dental professionals can better predict the outcomes of intentional replantation and provide their patients with informed, realistic expectations for their treatment.

## 10.3 Transplantation

Transplantation in dentistry is a sophisticated procedure that involves relocating a tooth from one location in the mouth to another, typically an extraction socket. This section introduces the concept, common scenarios, and critical factors influencing the success of transplantation. Transplantation is defined as the process of moving a tooth from one location in the mouth and implanting it into an extraction socket. A prevalent scenario for this procedure involves using the mandibular or maxillary third molars, often referred to as wisdom teeth, to replace a first molar that requires extraction. The need for such a replacement could arise due to various reasons, most commonly caries or fracture of the first molar [7, 8].

One of the most crucial aspects of a successful transplantation is maintaining the vitality of the periodontal ligament and cementum. These structures are essential for the reattachment of the tooth in its new location and play a significant role in the tooth's functionality post-surgery. The periodontal ligament contains the cells necessary for the tooth to integrate into its new position, while the cementum is vital for the attachment of these ligaments to the tooth. During the transplantation surgery, it is paramount to avoid direct damage to the transplanted tooth, especially the periodontal ligament and cementum. Any harm to these structures can significantly hinder the reattachment of the periodontal ligament and, consequently, the overall success of the transplantation. The surgical technique should be meticulously planned and executed to ensure the integrity of the tooth and its supporting structures.

The degree of root apex formation in the transplanted tooth is a critical factor in the success of transplantation. It is well-established that teeth with incomplete root formation have a higher success rate in terms of preservation and vitality maintenance of the pulp compared to teeth with completely formed roots. Incomplete root formation allows for continued development and revascularization of the pulp, enhancing the tooth's ability to integrate and function normally in its new location. Dental transplantation is a complex procedure requiring careful consideration of various factors. The vitality of the periodontal ligament and cementum, meticulous surgical technique to avoid direct damage, and the degree of root apex formation all play pivotal roles in the success of the transplantation. By understanding and addressing these factors, dental professionals can enhance the likelihood of a favorable outcome, providing patients with a functional and natural-looking replacement for extracted teeth. As we delve deeper into this topic, we will explore the detailed methodologies, patient selection criteria, and postoperative care essential to the successful execution of dental transplantation.

1. Indication

   Successful dental transplantation hinges on the meticulous selection of appropriate cases. This section delves into the crucial criteria and conditions that need to be met for a favorable prognosis in dental transplantation.

   (a) Availability of a nonfunctioning donor tooth:

      The primary prerequisite for transplantation is the availability of a nonfunctioning tooth that can serve as a donor. This typically involves a tooth that is not essential for the patient's current dental function or aesthetic, such as a wisdom tooth. The donor tooth should be in a healthy condition, free from caries or periodontal disease, to ensure the best chance of successful transplantation.

   (b) Suitable mesiodistal width:

      The mesiodistal width of the donor tooth must be compatible with the recipient site. This ensures that the transplanted tooth fits appropriately within the space and aligns correctly with adjacent teeth. A mismatch in size could lead to complications, including improper occlusion, aesthetic issues, or increased susceptibility to periodontal problems.

   (c) Recipient site conditions:

      The site where the tooth will be transplanted must be conducive to the procedure. This means it should be free of inflammation and bone destruction. A healthy recipient site is critical as it provides a stable and infection-free foundation for the transplanted tooth to integrate and function. Any signs of periodontal disease or ongoing infection must be addressed before the transplantation.

(d) Stage of root formation:

The most suitable teeth for transplantation are those with approximately two-thirds of the root formed. Teeth at this stage of development have a higher likelihood of successful pulp revascularization and continued root development once transplanted. This is crucial for the long-term viability and stability of the tooth. When transplanting a tooth with a fully formed root, the chances of revascularization decrease, and endodontic treatment may be required after transplantation to address this issue [9, 10].

The selection of appropriate cases for dental transplantation is vital for its success. A thorough assessment of the donor tooth's health, size compatibility, recipient site condition, and the developmental stage of the tooth's root is imperative (Fig. 10.3). By carefully considering these factors, dental professionals can significantly enhance the prognosis of dental transplantation, ensuring the transplanted tooth functions effectively and integrates harmoniously within the patient's dentition. As we move forward, we will explore the surgical techniques, postoperative care, and long-term management strategies that are integral to the success of dental transplantation.

2. Surgical Procedure

The surgical process for dental transplantation is a systematic approach aimed at relocating a healthy, nonfunctional tooth to a site where it is needed. This section provides a step-by-step guide to the procedure, highlighting the essential stages for a successful transplantation.

(a) Presurgical preparation:

Prior to the surgery, it is imperative to ensure the oral environment is conducive to a successful transplantation. This involves caries control and periodontal treatment around the surgical area to address any existing dental issues and minimize the risk of postoperative complications.

(b) Disinfection of the surgical site:

The surgical site, both where the tooth will be extracted and where it will be transplanted, should be thoroughly disinfected using iodine or chlorhexidine. This step is crucial for reducing the risk of infection during and after the procedure.

(c) Local anesthesia:

To ensure patient comfort and a pain-free experience, local anesthesia is administered to the area surrounding both the donor and recipient sites.

(d) Preparation of the recipient site:

If the recipient site does not have an existing extraction socket, an artificial alveolus is created using an implant drill. This provides a space for the donor tooth to be placed. If a tooth is being replaced, it is carefully extracted to prepare the site for transplantation.

(e) Extraction of the donor tooth:

The donor tooth is carefully extracted, ensuring minimal damage to the tooth

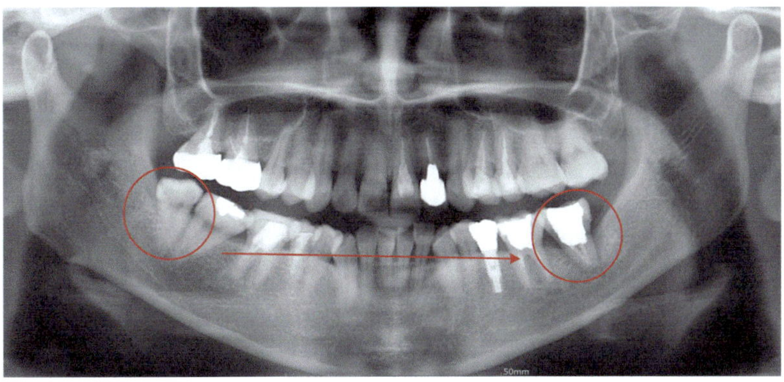

**Fig. 10.3** Preoperative panoramic view. Transplantation of right third molar to left second molar site (by Courtesy of prof. Son SA)

and its surrounding structures, particularly the periodontal ligament and cementum, which are crucial for reintegration.

(f) Apicoectomy and retrograde filling (if necessary):

In cases where the donor tooth has a fully formed root, an apicoectomy is performed, and a retrograde filling using mineral trioxide aggregate (MTA) is placed. This is essential to prevent potential infection and ensure the health of the tooth posttransplantation.

(g) Placement and fixation of the transplanted tooth:

The donor tooth is then placed into the recipient site. It is carefully positioned and secured using suturing, ensuring proper alignment and stability. Any occlusal interference is eliminated to prevent undue stress on the tooth during healing.

(h) Postoperative care:

Stitches are typically removed approximately 2 weeks after the surgery. For the first week post-surgery, a liquid diet is recommended to minimize stress on the transplanted tooth. The area should be gently cleaned using chlorhexidine to prevent infection.

(i) Diet and occlusal stress management:

As the retention of transplanted teeth can be weaker than natural teeth, it is important to avoid occlusal stress. A normal diet can usually be resumed about 6 weeks after the surgery, once the tooth has had sufficient time to integrate.

(j) Endodontic treatment for complete roots:

In cases where the transplanted tooth has a fully formed root, endodontic treatment is typically required. This should be performed about 1 month after the surgery to ensure the pulp is healthy and to prevent any potential infection (Fig. 10.4).

In conclusion, the surgical procedure for dental transplantation is a complex process that requires careful planning, precise execution, and diligent postoperative care. Each step, from the initial preparation to the post-surgery management, plays a vital role in the success of the transplantation (Fig. 10.5). By adhering to these guidelines, dental professionals can significantly enhance the outcome of the procedure, providing patients with a functional and aesthetically pleasing solution for missing or damaged teeth. As we move forward, we will explore the long-term management and potential complications associated with dental transplantation.

3. Prognosis

The prognosis of dental transplantation depends on a variety of factors, including the precision of surgical technique, appropriate case selection, and postoperative care. This section provides an overview of what to expect following a dental transplantation, highlighting both the successes and potential complications.

(a) Long-term maintenance:

When performed with meticulous attention to detail and appropriate case selection, dental transplantation can maintain the transplanted tooth without root resorption for over 5 years. This longevity is contingent upon swift and accurate execution during surgery, as well as diligent postoperative care. The aim is to ensure that the periodontal ligament and cementum remain vital, which is essential for the long-term integration and function of the tooth.

(b) Criteria for success and failure:

Typically, the success of a transplanted tooth is evaluated over time. If the transplanted tooth is lost within the first year, it is generally considered a failure. This early loss can be due to several factors, including failure of the tooth to integrate, infection, or damage to the periodontal ligament during the procedure. A successful transplantation, conversely, is one where the tooth remains functional, aesthetically pleasing, and free of resorption for several years postoperation.

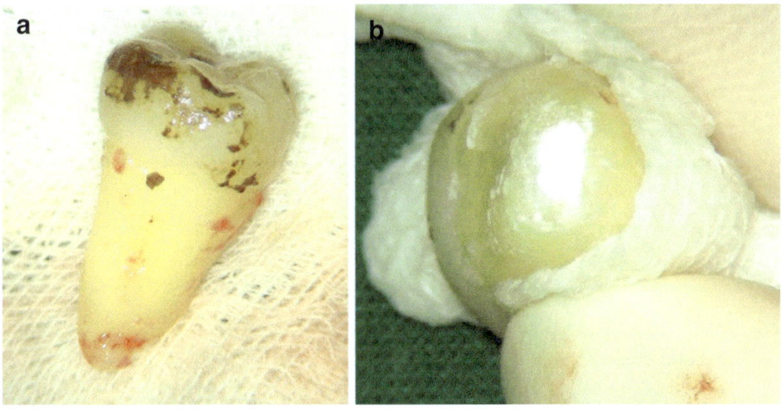

**Fig. 10.4** Intraoperative photo. (**a**) Extracted right mandibular third molar (**b**) apicoectomy and retrograde filling using MTA

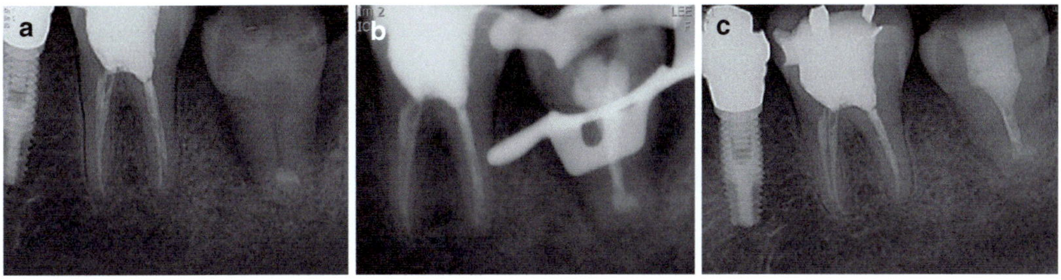

**Fig. 10.5** X-ray view after transplantation. (**a**) Immediate after replantation, (**b**) 6 weeks after replantation, (**c**) 6 months after replantation

(c) Root canal treatment and ankylosis:

Root canal treatment of the transplanted tooth, particularly those with fully formed roots, can lead to ankylosis—the fusion of the tooth to the bone. This condition is often accompanied by root resorption. However, it's important to note that this resorption typically progresses very slowly. Even in cases where ankylosis and resorption occur, the transplanted tooth can often continue to perform its functional and aesthetic roles for several years.

(d) Clinical value of transplantation:

Despite the potential complications, dental transplantation remains a clinically valuable procedure. When successful, it offers a natural-looking and functional solution for missing or damaged teeth. Moreover, even in cases where complications arise, such as slow-progressing root resorption, the transplanted tooth can often continue to serve the patient well for many years.

The prognosis of dental transplantation is generally favorable, provided that the procedure is carried out with precision, careful planning, and appropriate case selection. While complications such as ankylosis and root resorption can occur, they often progress slowly and do not immediately compromise the function and aesthetics of the transplanted tooth. Regular follow-ups and diligent oral care are essential for monitoring the health of the transplanted tooth and addressing any issues as they arise. By understanding the potential outcomes and maintaining a proactive approach to care, patients and dental professionals can work together to achieve a long-lasting and successful result from dental transplantation (Fig. 10.6).

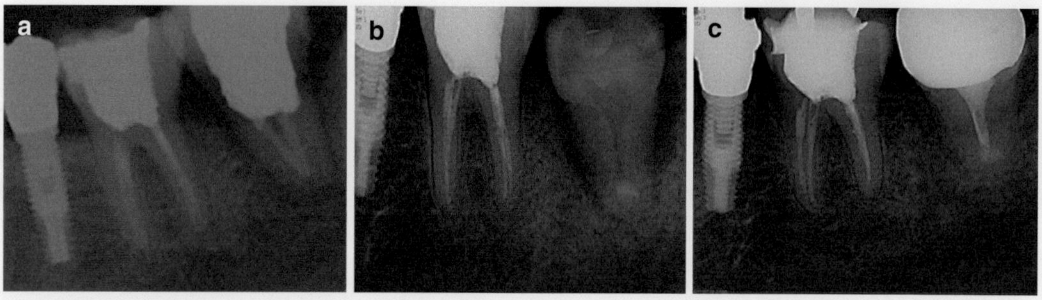

**Fig. 10.6** X-ray view before and after transplantation. (**a**) Preoperative view, (**b**) immediate after replantation, (**c**) 6 months after replantation

## 10.4 Conclusion

This chapter has examined the indications, surgical processes, and prognosis of the two types of autotransplantation—replantation and transplantation. Considering their clinical utility, it can be said that these procedures are valuable techniques.

## References

1. Cha IH, Yu JH, Lee JH, et al. Textbook of oral and maxillofacial surgery. 4th ed. Koonja Publisher; 2023. p. 108–10.
2. Tsukiboshi M. Autotransplantation of teeth. Quintessence publishing Co.; 2001.
3. Andreasen JO. The effect of splinting upon periodontal healing after replantation of permanent incisors in monkeys. Acta Odontol Scand. 1975;33:313–23. https://www.tandfonline.com/doi/abs/10.3109/00016357509004636
4. Galanter DR, Minami RT. The periodontal status of autografted teeth. A pilot study of thirty-one cases. Oral Surg Oral Med Oral Pathol. 1968;26:145–59. https://doi.org/10.1016/0030-4220(68)90243-0.
5. Andreasen JO, Hjorting-Hansen E, Jolst O. A clinical and radiographic study of 76 autotransplanted third molars. Scand J Dent Res. 1970;78:512–23. https://doi.org/10.1111/j.1600-0722.1970.tb02104.x.
6. Schwartz O, Bergmann P, Klausen B. Resortption of autotransplanted human teeth: a retrospective study of 291 transplantations over a period of 25 years. Int Endod J. 1985;18(2):119–31. https://doi.org/10.1111/j.1365-2591.1985.tb00428.x.
7. Andreasen JO. Autotransplantation of molars. In: Andreasen JO, editor. Atlas of replantation and transplantation of teeth. Copenhagen: Munksgaard; 1990. p. 111–38.
8. Nordenram A. Autotransplantation of teeth. A clinical and experimental investigation. Acta Odontol Scand. 1963;21(33):7–26.
9. Andreasen JO, Paulsen HU, Yu Z, et al. A long-term study of 379 autotransplanted premolars. Part I. Surgical procedures and standardized techniques for monitoring healing. Eur J Orthod. 1990;12:3–13. https://doi.org/10.1093/ejo/12.1.3.
10. Andresen JO, Paulsen HU, Yu Z, et al. A long-term study of 370 autotransplanted premolar. Part III. Periodontal healing subsequent to transplantation. Eur J Orthod. 1990;12(1):25–37. https://doi.org/10.1093/ejo/12.1.25.

# 11 Innovations and Future Trends in Tooth Extraction

## Contents



## 11.1 Introduction

Tooth extraction, a cornerstone of dental practice, has evolved remarkably from its rudimentary origins to a sophisticated interplay of science and technology [1]. Historically, extractions were primitive, often performed by non-specialists with minimal tools and understanding of oral anatomy. This history contrasts sharply with today's precise, patient-centric procedures that emphasize minimal invasiveness and maximal preservation [2].

Central to modern extraction practices is the preservation of alveolar bone—a critical factor in post-extraction healing and subsequent dental restorations like implants [2]. Equally important is the prevention of nerve injuries, a challenge that continues to inspire innovative solutions in dental surgery [3]. These considerations have transformed tooth extraction from a mere removal procedure to a nuanced art that balances immediate needs with long-term oral health outcomes.

Moreover, the novel utilization of extracted teeth as graft material marks a significant stride toward sustainable, biocompatible dental practices [4]. These teeth, once considered medical waste, are now being repurposed, showcasing dentistry's commitment to innovation and environmental consciousness [5].

This chapter aims to provide a comprehensive exploration of these facets. We will journey through the historical evolution of tooth extraction, explore the contemporary practices focusing on alveolar bone preservation and nerve



S.-G. Kim et al., *Advanced Strategies for Tooth Extraction in Dentistry*,
https://doi.org/10.1007/978-981-97-6532-4_11

injury prevention, and highlight the innovative use of extracted teeth in dental grafting. Each section is designed to offer insights into the current state, emerging trends, and future directions, culminating in a synthesis of how these developments are reshaping the landscape of dental surgery.

## 11.2 Current Practices and Challenges in Tooth Extraction

Tooth extraction, although a commonly performed procedure in dental practice, presents a multitude of intricacies and obstacles. The conventional methods of extraction predominantly rely on the utilization of forceps and elevators, with the main emphasis being on the mechanical extraction of the tooth. While these techniques have proven to be effective, the level of complexity involved can significantly differ depending on various factors such as the position of the tooth, the morphology of its roots, and patient-specific anatomical considerations.

The success of a tooth extraction procedure relies on the dentist's proficiency in understanding and navigating through these complexities. Factors such as the angulation and depth of tooth roots, the presence of bony obstacles, and the proximity of vital structures can substantially influence the level of difficulty in extracting a tooth [6]. For instance, impacted wisdom teeth, which often require surgical removal, may involve intricate techniques such as sectioning the tooth into smaller fragments or removing a portion of the surrounding bone to facilitate extraction.

Additionally, the individual characteristics of each patient must also be considered when planning an extraction [7]. Anatomical variations, such as the proximity of nerves or sinuses, may necessitate additional caution and precision during the procedure. Furthermore, medical conditions or medications taken by the patient can also impact the extraction process, requiring careful consideration to ensure patient safety and optimal outcomes [8].

Advancements in dental technology and surgical techniques have revolutionized tooth extraction procedures in recent years. Dentists now have access to alternative approaches that aim to reduce the invasiveness and associated risks of traditional extraction methods, while still ensuring the successful removal of the tooth. These new techniques, such as minimally invasive procedures [9] and the use of lasers [10], have shifted the paradigm of tooth extraction toward a more patient-friendly and precise approach. One of the key advancements in tooth extraction is the development of minimally invasive procedures. These techniques involve smaller incisions and less tissue removal, minimizing trauma to surrounding structures [9]. Minimally invasive approaches also result in reduced postoperative pain, bleeding, and swelling, leading to faster recovery times for patients. These procedures employ specialized tools and instruments, designed to navigate, and remove the tooth with minimal disruption to the surrounding tissues.

The utilization of lasers in tooth extraction is another significant advancement in the field of dentistry [10]. Lasers offer several advantages, including improved precision, reduced bleeding, and decreased postoperative discomfort. Laser technology allows dentists to precisely target and remove the tooth, while simultaneously sealing blood vessels and nerve endings, resulting in a more controlled and less traumatic extraction. Furthermore, lasers have the unique capability to promote tissue regeneration and reduce the risk of infection, thereby enhancing the overall healing process [11].

One of the main hurdles in removing teeth is safeguarding the alveolar bone and avoiding harm to nerves. The close location of the area where the tooth is removed to essential body parts, like the inferior alveolar nerve (IAN), requires meticulous planning and precise surgical methods. Advances in both imaging technology and surgical approaches are focused on reducing the possibility of nerve injury while maintaining the strength of the bone, which is vital for any future dental procedures. Using orthodontic force can create a gap between the root tip and the IAN [12]. Additionally, a technique known as coronectomy is often employed to prevent damage to the IAN [13].

The utilization of extracted teeth as graft material presents an innovative approach in regenerative dentistry [14]. Targeting specifically the dentin within these extracted teeth, this concept offers numerous advantages, such as reducing medical waste and capitalizing on the biocompatibility and structural similarities between dentin and natural bone. By repurposing extracted teeth as bone grafts, the field of dentistry can significantly minimize waste generation and contribute to sustainable healthcare practices [15]. Each aspect of this section underscores the ongoing evolution in tooth extraction methodologies, balancing the need for effective removal with the broader objectives of patient safety, procedural success, and sustainable practices.

## 11.3 Preventing Nerve Injury and Promoting Bone Health

### 11.3.1 Coronectomy

Coronectomy, an innovative dental procedure, is gaining prominence as a safer alternative to traditional tooth extraction, especially in cases where there is a high risk of nerve injury [13]. This technique is particularly relevant in the removal of impacted third molars, where the proximity of the roots to the IAN presents a significant risk of nerve damage [16].

The procedure of coronectomy involves the deliberate retention of the tooth root while removing only the crown. If enamel is remained after coronectomy, the infection risk is increased [17]. Accordingly, precise resection of crown is required (Fig. 11.1). The technique begins with a careful incision and flap elevation to expose the tooth. The crown is then separated from the roots using precise dental instruments, ensuring minimal disturbance to the surrounding bone and nerve structures. Using 3D-drilled sleeve, the precision of the procedure can be improved [16]. The roots, which are left in situ, are typically covered with a bone grafting material to promote bone health and healing. Some roots can be migrated and the distance is 2.33–3.43 mm at 6 months postoperatively [18, 19]. The velocity of migration is gradually decreased and stopped at 12 months postoperatively [18].

Coronectomy is particularly indicated in patients where the tooth roots are near the IAN, as identified through radiographic imaging (Fig. 11.2). It is a preferred option in cases where traditional extraction methods pose a high risk of nerve damage, which can lead to numbness or altered sensation in the lower lip and chin. The primary advantage of coronectomy is the significantly reduced risk of nerve injury. Coronectomy significantly reduced the risk of IAN injury (odds ratio [OR]: 0.14), postoperative pain (OR: 0.97), and alveolitis (OR: 0.38) compared to complete extraction [13]. By preserving the tooth roots, this technique also helps in maintaining bone integrity and health, especially in the mandibular region. This is crucial for future dental interventions, such as dental implants, and overall oral health.

Postoperative care is crucial in coronectomy. Patients are advised to maintain oral hygiene to prevent infection. Coronectomy also showed an increased risk of surgical reintervention (OR: 5.38) [13]. Regular follow-ups are necessary to monitor the health of the retained roots and surrounding bone. In some cases, the roots may migrate or resorb over time, further reducing the risk of nerve damage. In 10-year follow-up study, only two subjects (4%) experienced complications, specifically root exposures, 8- or 9-years post-surgery [20]. When compared to complete removal of mandibular third molars, less incidences of bleeding and dry socket are observed in the coronectomy group [21]. IAN deficit is significantly higher in the complete removal group (3.7%) compared to the coronectomy group (0.5%) [21]. Though there was no permanent nerve injury after coronectomy, other systematic review reported that transient IAN injury was in 0–2.20% of successful coronectomy and 0–8% of failed coronectomy [18]. Coronectomy can reduce the risk of nerve injury by 84% [22].

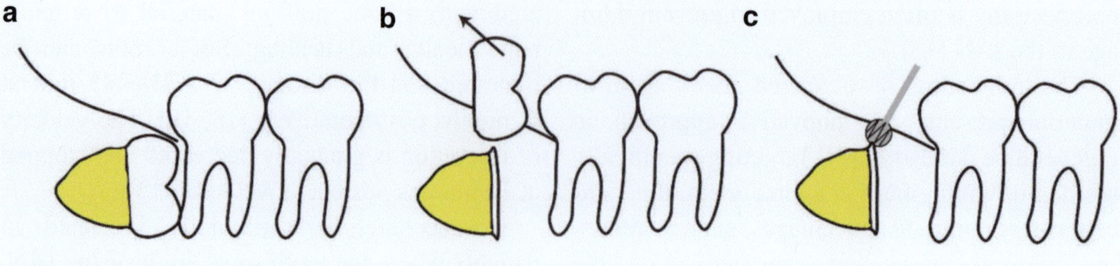


**Fig. 11.1** Procedure for the coronectomy. (**a**) Impacted tooth should be exposed, (**b**) crown portion of impacted tooth is removed first, (**c**) the remained enamel should be removed for the prevention of potential complications

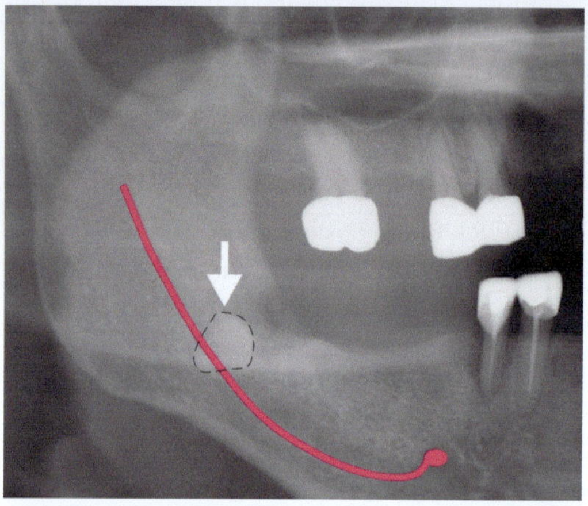

**Fig. 11.2** Coronectomy performed on an impacted third molar (arrow) in close proximity to IAN (red)

As coronectomy is the procedure of removing tooth crown, the pulp tissue will be exposed after coronectomy. When compared coronectomy with concurrent root canal treatment (RCT) to that without, the frequency of postoperative infection is 87.5% with RCT and 12.5% without RCT [23]. Coronectomy represents a significant advancement in oral surgery, aligning with the goals of preventing nerve injury and promoting bone health. As dental professionals continue to seek safer and more effective tooth extraction methods, coronectomy offers a promising approach, particularly in complex cases where nerve damage is a primary concern. However, Fraser cautions against the unnecessary use of coronectomy in cases with a low risk of nerve damage, highlighting the potential for increased surgical risks and future complications when the procedure is not judiciously indicated [24].

### 11.3.2 Orthodontic Tooth Movement

Orthodontic tooth movement is an innovative approach utilized in the extraction of mandibular third molars, or wisdom teeth, to mitigate the risk of nerve damage [25]. This technique involves applying orthodontic forces to the tooth prior to extraction, aiming to reposition it in a manner that minimizes the potential harm to nearby nerves [26].

The extraction of lower wisdom teeth poses a risk to the IAN, located close to the roots of these teeth. Damage to this nerve during extraction can lead to numbness or altered sensation in the lower lip and chin, a complication with potentially long-term effects. By employing orthodontic forces to strategically move the tooth away from this nerve, the risk of such nerve injuries is significantly reduced [27].

In standard orthodontic treatments, excessive force can lead to root resorption, where the tooth's root structure is gradually eroded. However, in the context of mandibular third molar extraction, this concern is secondary. Since the tooth is destined for removal, the primary focus shifts to maneuvering it safely for extraction, rendering the risk of root resorption less relevant. The process involves applying orthodontic forces over a period, using braces or other devices, to reposition the tooth [27]. This pre-extraction movement is designed to ensure that when the time for extraction arrives, the procedure is less complicated and the risk to the nerve is minimized [28]. This approach is particularly advantageous in cases where the tooth is near the nerve or in complex extraction scenarios.

The initial diagnosis of the proximity of a tooth to the mandibular canal is determined through radiographic evaluations and predetermined criteria [29]. These assessments focus on radiologic characteristics that suggest a probable closeness of the root to IAN. Depending on the level of impaction, the surgical procedures adopted can vary significantly. In cases of superficial semi-impactions, a direct bracket attachment may suffice [27]. However, for more deeply impacted teeth, more invasive techniques are necessary, such as the elevation of a full-thickness mucoperiosteal flap and osteotomy [27].

Orthodontic mechanotherapy, the approach used to facilitate this process, can vary in technique. Three primary biomechanical methods are commonly employed: firstly, attaching simple cantilever to the lower third molar (M3) buttonhole (Fig. 11.3a); secondly, using the posterior maxillary region as an anchor for the orthodontic extrusion of M3 (Fig. 11.3b); and thirdly, connecting cantilever springs to a bonded orthodontic bracket on the M3, supplemented with a multiple-loop spring wire for the tooth's distal movement. A specific technique within these methods involves using a 0.016-inch nickel and titanium (NiTi) wire for leveling the M3. This is followed by active extrusion with a 0.016–0.022-inch stainless steel spring wire, which leverages a miniscrew attached to the second premolar and first molar for maximum skeletal anchorage [27].

This orthodontic approach significantly reduces the likelihood of nerve-related complications, a crucial concern given the potential for long-term consequences [26, 27]. However, the success of this method hinges on detailed planning and a collaborative effort between the orthodontist and oral surgeon. The decision to use orthodontic movement is based on a comprehensive assessment of each individual case, ensuring that the treatment is specifically tailored to meet the unique needs and risks involved. While not a universal solution for all wisdom tooth extractions, orthodontic tooth movement presents a valuable option in cases with a heightened risk of nerve damage. It exemplifies the importance of personalized care in dental treatments, prioritizing patient safety and long-term wellbeing in complex dental procedures.

### 11.3.3 Ridge Preservation Technique

Ridge preservation, a pivotal concept in modern dental surgery, pertains to the array of procedures and techniques employed to conserve the alveolar ridge's structure and integrity following tooth extraction [30]. The primary purpose of ridge preservation is to maintain the natural contour and density of the alveolar bone, which is crucial for future dental restorative procedures, such as dental implants or bridges. This practice is particularly significant because, following tooth extraction, the alveolar ridge tends to undergo resorption, leading to a loss in both vertical height and horizontal width of the bone [31]. Such bone loss can complicate, or even preclude, subsequent dental restorations while also affecting the aesthetic and functional aspects of the oral cavity.

Historically, the significance of ridge preservation was recognized as dental practitioners observed the natural consequences of tooth loss [30]. Initially, the focus was primarily on immediate restorative solutions without much consideration for the long-term structural changes in the jawbone. However, as the field of oral surgery and dentistry evolved, the understanding of alveolar bone dynamics post-extraction deepened [31]. Researchers and clinicians noticed the pattern of bone degradation that followed extractions, sparking interest in developing methods to counteract this process [30].

The evolution of ridge preservation techniques is marked by a transition from merely reactive to proactive strategies [32]. Early approaches were rudimentary, often involving simple socket fillings with various materials to encourage bone retention. As the field progressed, these techniques became more sophisticated, incorporating advanced biomaterials and methodologies. These included the use of bone grafts, growth factors, and barrier membranes, each playing a distinct role in supporting and stimulating the natural bone healing process [30].

This historical journey of ridge preservation reflects a broader shift in dental practice: from a focus on problem resolution to a preventative, holistic approach that considers long-term oral

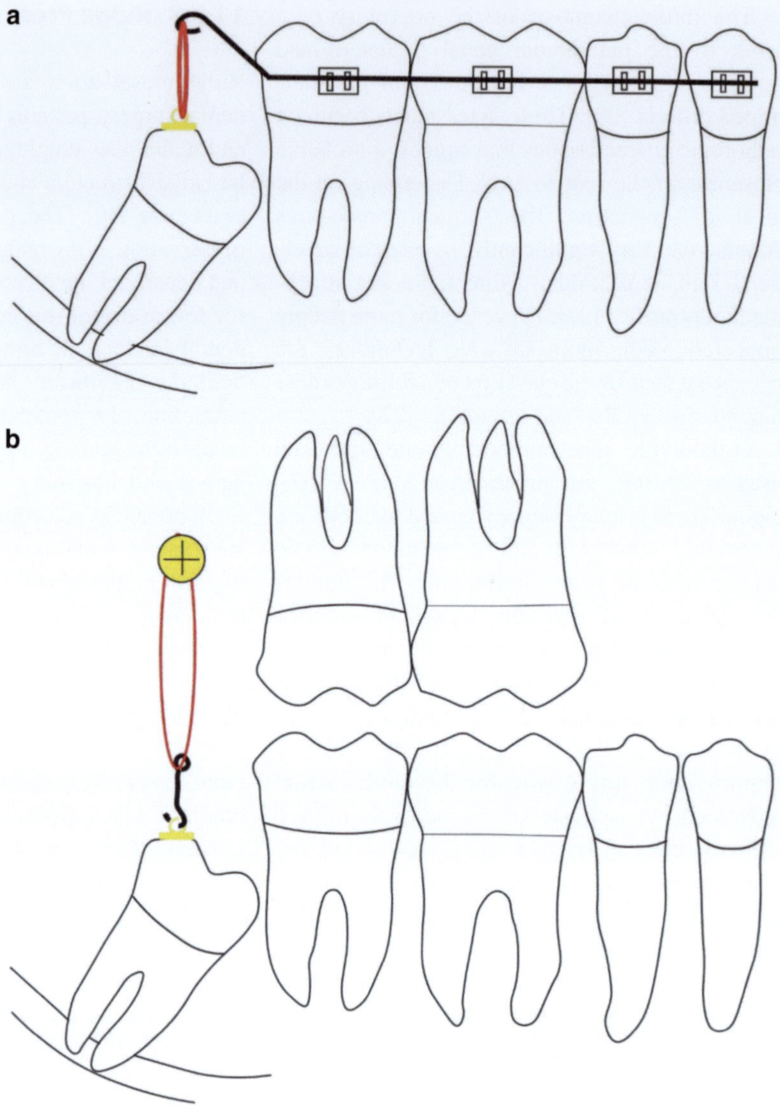


**Fig. 11.3** Orthodontic force application for the traction of impacted third molar. (**a**) Orthodontic appliances can be used for the traction of impacted tooth, (**b**) the screw anchorage system for the traction of impacted tooth

health outcomes. This paradigm shift underscores the importance of maintaining jawbone integrity, not only for immediate functional and aesthetic needs but also for future dental interventions. As we continue to explore the intricacies of ridge preservation, this practice has become an integral component of modern dental care, reflecting a deep understanding of oral physiology and a commitment to preserving the natural structure of the mouth for long-term health and wellness.

Post-extraction, the alveolar ridge is subject to a natural resorption process, where the bone that previously supported the tooth begins to diminish both in volume and density [32]. This phenomenon is most pronounced within the first few months following an extraction. If unchecked, this resorption can lead to significant structural changes in the jawbone, compromising the integrity and shape of the oral cavity [30]. Preserving the alveolar ridge is critical for several reasons. Structurally, it maintains the jawbone's shape, which is essential for facial aesthetics. Loss of bone can lead to a sunken appearance around the mouth, significantly altering one's facial profile. Functionally, the ridge serves as the foundation for any future dental prostheses. A well-preserved ridge ensures that options like implants can be securely anchored, providing a stable and durable solution that mimics the natural function of real teeth.

The state of the alveolar ridge post-extraction directly influences the range and success of restorative dental options available to a patient. A well-preserved ridge offers a robust foundation for dental implants, which are increasingly popular due to their natural appearance and functionality. Implants require sufficient bone for placement, and a diminished alveolar ridge can necessitate additional procedures like bone grafting, complicating, and prolonging the treatment process. Furthermore, a preserved ridge aids in maintaining proper alignment and spacing of the remaining teeth. When the ridge deteriorates, adjacent teeth can shift, leading to misalignment issues that affect bite, chewing efficiency, and even speech. These shifts can also create spaces that are difficult to clean, escalating the risk of periodontal disease and tooth decay.

The field of dental surgery has seen significant advancements in the techniques for ridge preservation, each designed to mitigate the effects of bone resorption following tooth extraction. These techniques vary in complexity, materials used, and suitability for different clinical scenarios (Fig. 11.4). The primary objective of all ridge preservation techniques is to maintain the volume

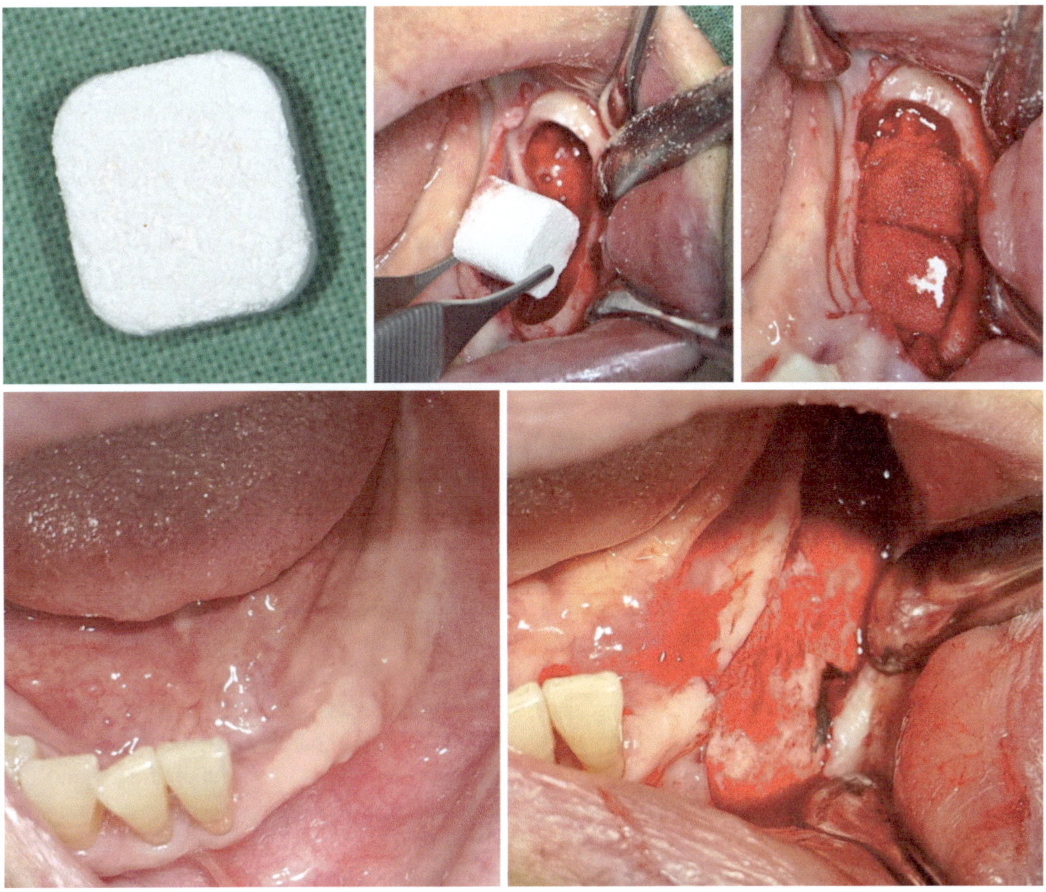

**Fig. 11.4** Using a combination graft of porcine-derived hydroxyapatite and type I collagen after tooth extraction. The grafts are prepped for placement into the alveolar ridge defect (upper row). Post blood absorption, the grafts turn red. One-month postoperation, the area is healing smoothly (lower left). Six months post-grafting, during implant installation, significant bone regeneration is observed in the alveolar ridge (lower right)

and structure of the alveolar ridge. The most common methods include as follows:

- Socket grafting: This technique involves placing a bone graft material directly into the extraction socket. The graft may be autograft (taken from the patient), allograft (donor bone), xenograft (animal bone), or alloplast (synthetic material). The choice depends on the specific case and patient preferences.
- Use of barrier membranes: Barrier membranes are often used in conjunction with grafting. They cover the graft material and extraction site, preventing soft tissue from invading the space and allowing the bone to regenerate more effectively.
- Growth factor application: This method involves applying growth factors, either alone or with other grafting materials, to stimulate bone growth and healing. These growth factors can be derived from the patient's blood (e.g., platelet-rich plasma—PRP) or synthetic sources.
- Flap management techniques: These are surgical techniques that involve manipulating the gum tissue around the extraction site to protect the bone graft and encourage proper healing.

There are several materials those can be considered for socket grafting materials (Table 11.1). Autografts offer excellent biocompatibility but require a second surgical site for harvesting the graft, which can increase patient discomfort and recovery time [33]. Allografts and xenografts eliminate the need for a second surgical site, but their integration with the patient's bone can vary. Allografts have a good track record of success [34], while xenografts, derived from animal sources, may take longer to integrate [35]. Alloplastic materials are synthetically created, offering a consistent quality, and avoiding potential issues with disease transmission. However, their integration with natural bone can be less predictable than biological grafts.

The results of the systematic review provide insightful data on the effectiveness of various grafting materials used in alveolar ridge preservation [36]. When allograft materials were used, the average horizontal ridge resorption was measured at $1.52 \pm 1.29$ mm. It was $1.47 \pm 0.92$ mm, $2.31 \pm 1.19$ mm, and $3.1 \pm 1.07$ mm for xenograft, alloplasts, and unassisted healing, respectively [36]. These results highlight the nuanced differences in the performance of various grafting materials in ridge preservation.

The choice between resorbable and non-resorbable membranes depends on the specific clinical situation (Table 11.2) [37]. Resorbable membranes, which dissolve over time, reduce the need for a second procedure to remove the membrane but may offer less protection to the graft material [38]. Non-resorbable membranes provide more robust protection but require a second surgery for removal [38].

The findings from a standard pairwise meta-analysis and a network meta-analysis (NMA) provide insightful comparisons regarding the effectiveness of various membranes in dental ridge preservation [39]. The analysis shows a significant advantage of resorbable membranes over the control group, with consistent findings across studies and no significant heterogeneity [39]. This advantage was evident regardless of whether the same graft material was used in both test and control groups, as seen in studies by Lim et al. [40] and Lekovic et al. [41]. Additionally, a comparison between crosslinked and non-crosslinked collagen membranes revealed a preference for non-crosslinked ones, attributed to their better biocompatibility despite the superior degradation resistance of crosslinked membranes [39]. The NMA further evaluated different coverage biomaterials, revealing a moderate to high reliability in comparisons, particularly between non-crosslinked resorbable membranes and the control group, and between crosslinked and non-crosslinked resorbable membranes. These results underscore the critical role of membrane selection in ridge preservation, emphasizing factors like biocompatibility, degradation resistance,

**Table 11.1** Socket grafting materials

| Type of graft | Source | Key characteristics | Considerations |
|---|---|---|---|
| Autograft | Patient's own body (e.g., chin, jaw, hip) | High biocompatibility, contains living cells for effective healing | Requires additional surgery site, increased recovery time |
| Allograft | Donor human bone (cadavers) | Eliminates need for second surgery site, good success rate | Low risk of immune reaction, processed to prevent disease transmission |
| Xenograft | Animal bone (commonly bovine or porcine) | Close mimicry to human bone, supports new bone growth | Slower integration, ethical/religious considerations for some patients |
| Alloplast | Synthetic materials (e.g., hydroxyapatite, calcium phosphates) | Consistent quality, no disease transmission risk | Less-predictable integration with natural bone, variety of materials with different outcomes |

**Table 11.2** Types of dental membranes for ridge preservation

| Type of membrane | Materials | Characteristics | Applications |
|---|---|---|---|
| Resorbable | Collagen, polylactic acid (PLA), polyglycolic acid (PGA), natural polymers | Biodegradable, absorbed by body over time, no need for removal surgery | Cases with minimal to moderate bone regeneration, low risk of membrane exposure |
| Non-Resorbable | ePTFE, dPTFE, titanium mesh, synthetic polymers | Stable, long-lasting, requires removal surgery | Complex cases with large bone defects or need for prolonged healing |

and exposure risk in clinical outcomes and decision-making [39].

Growth factors can significantly enhance healing and bone formation [42]. Their use, however, often involves more complex preparation and handling, and the cost can be higher compared to traditional grafting materials. These techniques are crucial in ensuring the stability of the graft material and proper healing of the site. However, they require a higher level of surgical skill and may increase the complexity of the procedure. In conclusion, the choice of ridge preservation technique is influenced by several factors, including the specific clinical scenario, patient health and preferences, cost considerations, and the expertise of the dental surgeon. Each method has its advantages and limitations, and often, a combination of techniques is employed to achieve the best outcome. The goal remains the same: to preserve the alveolar ridge's structure for future restorative dentistry and to maintain the patient's oral health and aesthetics.

## 11.4 Using Extracted Teeth as Graft Material

In Melvin L. Morris's 1967 paper, the effects of decalcified human tooth roots on rat tissues were explored. Decalcification with 5% ethylenediaminetetraacetic acid was found to reduce the inductive influence of cementum and dentin, a contrast to undecalcified implants [43]. Morris's subsequent works [44–46] further revealed the significant role of the physical state of tooth materials in their interaction with tissues, showing how both preserved and decalcified materials influence bone and marrow growth. While preserved material led to bone-root fusions and marrow ossicles, decalcified material hastened the formation of marrow-containing ossicles [45, 46]. These findings underpin the rationale for autologous tooth grafts, suggesting their potential in stimulating cellular activities and bone formation.

The first human application of autologous dentin grafts began in 2011 [47], leading to various studies investigating their effectiveness in oral and maxillofacial surgeries [48–50]. A review paper analyzing 81 studies, including these clinical applications, highlights autogenous demineralized dentin as a potential bone graft substitute [51]. Eleven studies with 215 patients showed that autogenous dentin is effective in maintaining bone volume, demonstrating promising results in histologic and histomorphometric analysis, and exhibiting a low complication rate [52].

The preparation of extracted teeth for grafting involves a meticulous process [53]. Initially, any soft tissues and pulp are removed from the extracted teeth. The roots are then cleaned to eliminate residual tissues, and small holes are created on the tooth surface to facilitate effective reagent penetration. The demineralization of the teeth is achieved using a vacuum-ultrasonic system in 0.6 N HCl for 90 min. After demineralization, the teeth are thoroughly washed and sterilized. The final step involves packaging these processed teeth in sterile tubes, ready for use as graft materials. This procedure ensures that the teeth are suitably prepared for effective grafting [53]. This is an example and there can be technical modifications (Fig. 11.5).

Nevertheless, the implementation of this approach requires careful consideration of several factors. Sterilization of the extracted teeth is crucial to eliminate any potential contaminants and ensure a safe grafting procedure [53]. Effective sterilization techniques should be selected to strike a balance between maintaining

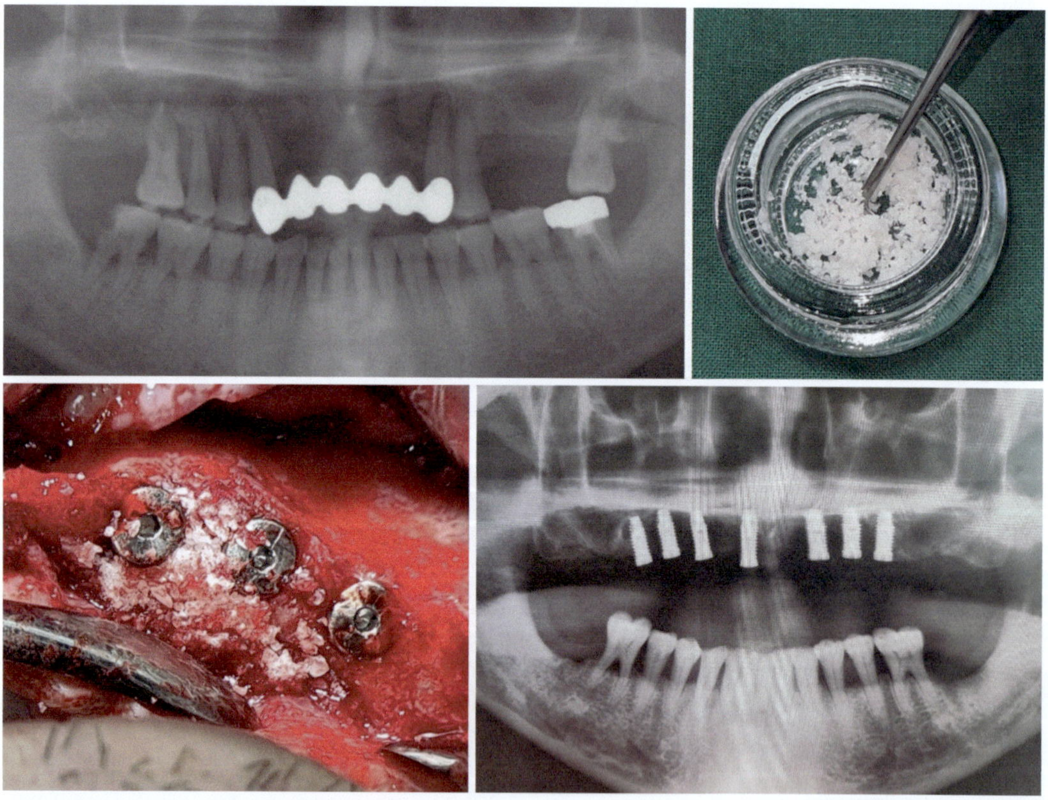

**Fig. 11.5** Utilizing extracted teeth as graft material for dental reconstruction. The initial stage showcases severe periodontitis in the maxillary teeth (upper left). After the extraction of all maxillary teeth, they are repurposed for an autologous dentin graft (upper right). For dental implantation, a combination graft incorporating this autologous dentin and additional material from the maxillary tuberosity is employed (lower left). The final image illustrates the successful implantation postoperatively (lower right)

the integrity of the dentin structure and eliminating any biohazardous components. Additionally, the composition of dentin as a graft material needs to be thoroughly evaluated to ensure compatibility with the surrounding tissues and promote successful bone regeneration [54]. This may involve optimizing the preparation and processing methods to retain the necessary biological and mechanical properties of dentin.

Autogenous tooth grafts show promising results in new bone formation after alveolar ridge preservation (ARP) procedures [52]. Histomorphometric examinations conducted between 4- and 7-months post-procedure revealed 20.78–66.5% new bone formation, surpassing the results of xenogeneic (20.6–36.5%) [55, 56] and allogeneic grafts (14–42%) [57]. Additionally, residual graft percentages for autogenous tooth grafts were lower (0.9–19.7%) compared to xenogeneic (19.0–36.6%) [56] and allogeneic (19–55%) [57] bone grafts, suggesting better resorption rates. This indicates that autogenous tooth grafts may be more efficient in bone regeneration and resorption compared to other materials [52].

When considering extracted teeth as graft material, it is crucial to evaluate each patient's unique circumstances. This includes assessing their overall health, anatomical factors, and the specific requirements of the grafting site. Additionally, the limited availability of autogenous dentin must be considered [53]. It is essential to determine if the extracted tooth grafts will suffice in terms of providing adequate support, integration, and functional restoration at the intended site.

## 11.5 Innovative Extraction Techniques

1. Powered Periotomes and Luxators in Atraumatic Tooth Extraction

   This technique minimizes alveolar bone loss and is beneficial for future or immediate implant placement. Using powered periotomes and luxators, precise tooth removal is achieved without raising mucoperiosteal flaps, reducing postoperative pain and preserving alveolar ridge dimensions [58].
2. Implant Drills for Tooth Extractions Prior to Immediate Implant Placement

   Implant drills thin root walls to enable atraumatic extractions, protecting surrounding bone structures. Tested on nine patients, this method has shown successful outcomes in immediate implant cases, with uneventful healing and effective osseointegration [59].
3. Piezosurgery in Tooth Extractions

   Piezosurgery offers precise, safe cuts in tooth extractions, sparing soft tissues and reducing nerve injury risks. It is especially effective in impacted tooth extractions, providing a more controlled approach and enhancing patient comfort and postoperative recovery [60].
4. Advancements in Hemostatic Materials for Dental Surgery

   A network meta-analysis evaluated different hemostatic agents for dental extraction in patients on oral antithrombotic therapy. Cyanoacrylate tissue adhesive and tranexamic acid were notably effective in reducing postoperative bleeding, outperforming conventional methods [61]. Hemostatic agents,

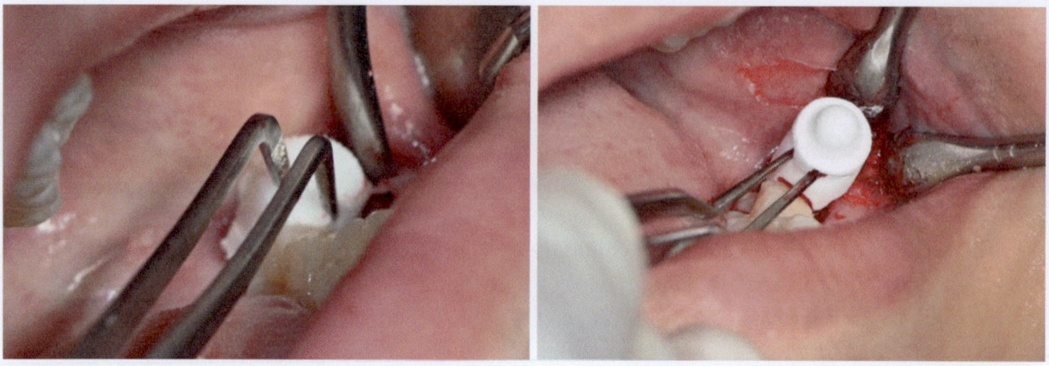

**Fig. 11.6** Applying hemostat in the extraction socket. A dental gelatin sponge is used for smaller sockets (left), while a collagen-based sponge suits larger sockets (right)

including natural and synthetic polymers, inorganic materials, and metal-containing materials, are utilized in various forms for wound care and surgeries (Fig. 11.6). Their development aims to improve safety and efficacy in controlling bleeding during dental surgeries [62].

## 11.6 Conclusion

In conclusion, this chapter underscores the remarkable progress in tooth extraction and grafting techniques. It acknowledges the pivotal role of sustainable practices in dentistry, highlighting the eco-friendly potential of using extracted teeth as graft material. Looking forward, the chapter anticipates further advancements and research in less invasive extraction methods, innovative grafting materials, and sustainable practices. This evolution in dental techniques aligns with the broader healthcare objectives of reducing patient discomfort, enhancing procedural efficiency, and promoting environmental responsibility in dental care.

## References

1. Udeabor SE, Heselich A, Al-Maawi S, Alqahtani AF, Sader R, Ghanaati S. Current knowledge on the healing of the extraction socket: a narrative review. Bioengineering. 2023;10:1145. https://doi.org/10.3390/bioengineering10101145.
2. Ucer C, Khan RS. Alveolar ridge preservation with autologous platelet-rich fibrin (PRF): case reports and the rationale. Dent J. 2023;11:244. https://doi.org/10.3390/dj11100244.
3. Li Y, Ling Z, Zhang H, et al. Association of the inferior alveolar nerve position and nerve injury: a systematic review and meta-analysis. Healthcare. 2022;10:1782. https://doi.org/10.3390/healthcare10091782.
4. Mahardawi B, Jiaranuchart S, Tompkins KA, Pimkhaokham A. Efficacy of the autogenous dentin graft for implant placement: a systematic review and meta-analysis of randomized controlled trials. Int J Oral Maxillofac Surg. 2023;52:604–12. https://doi.org/10.1016/j.ijom.2022.10.014.
5. Kim YK, Lee J, Um IW, et al. Tooth-derived bone graft material. J Korean Assoc Oral Maxillofac Surg. 2013;39:103–11. https://doi.org/10.5125/jkaoms.2013.39.3.103.
6. Astramskaitė I, Poškevičius L, Juodžbalys G. Factors determining tooth extraction anxiety and fear in adult dental patients: a systematic review. Int J Oral Maxillofac Surg. 2016;45:1630–43. https://doi.org/10.1016/j.ijom.2016.06.019.
7. Duarte-Rodrigues L, Miranda EFP, Souza TO, de Paiva HN, Falci SGM, Galvão EL. Third molar removal and its impact on quality of life: systematic review and meta-analysis. Qual Life Res. 2018;27:2477–89. https://doi.org/10.1007/s11136-018-1889-1.
8. Slavkin HC, Dubois PA, Kleinman DV, Fuccillo R. Science-informed health policies for oral and systemic health. J Healthc Leadersh. 2023;15:43–57. https://doi.org/10.2147/JHL.S363657.
9. Bin Rubaia'an MA, Alotaibi MK, Neyaz AA. A minimally invasive technique for the retrieval of fractured root tips. Cureus. 2023;15:e41458. https://doi.org/10.7759/cureus.41458.
10. Nunes CEN, Andrade KDS, Martins CA, Chaves FN, Oliveira DHIP, Sampieri MBDS. Effectiveness of low power laser in reducing postoperative signs and symptoms after third molar surgery: a triple-blind clinical trial. Braz Dent J. 2023;34:158–68. https://doi.org/10.1590/0103-6440202305413.

11. Han Y, Zhu J, Hu S, Li C, Zhang X. Nd:YAG laser therapy on postoperative pain, swelling, and trismus after mandibular third molar surgery: a randomized double-blinded clinical study. Lasers Med Sci. 2023;38:176. https://doi.org/10.1007/s10103-023-03836-9.
12. Zhou J, Hong H, Zhou H, et al. Orthodontic extraction of a high-risk impacted mandibular third molar contacting the inferior alveolar nerve, with the aid of a ramus mini-screw. Quintessence Int. 2021;52:538–46. https://doi.org/10.3290/j.qi.b1244345.
13. Peixoto AO, Bachesk AB, Leal MOCD, et al. Benefits of coronectomy in lower third molar surgery: a systematic review and meta-analysis. J Oral Maxillofac Surg. 2024;82(1):73–92. https://doi.org/10.1016/j.joms.2023.09.024.
14. Xu X, Peng D, Zhou B, et al. Demineralized dentin matrix promotes gingival healing in alveolar ridge preservation of premolars extracted for orthodontic reason: a split-mouth study. Front Endocrinol. 2023;14:1281649. https://doi.org/10.3389/fendo.2023.1281649.
15. Mahardawi B, Kyaw TT, Mattheos N, Pimkhaokham A. The clinical efficacy of autogenous dentin blocks prepared chairside for alveolar ridge augmentation: a systematic review and meta-analysis. Clin Oral Implants Res. 2023;34:1025–37. https://doi.org/10.1111/clr.14131.
16. Pacheco A, Soós B, Lempel E, et al. The effect of individual drilling sleeves on the precision of coronectomy tooth sections. An in vitro 3D-printed jaw model experiment. Clin Oral Investig. 2023;27:6769–80. https://doi.org/10.1007/s00784-023-05289-4.
17. Frenkel B, Givol N, Shoshani Y. Coronectomy of the mandibular third molar: a retrospective study of 185 procedures and the decision to repeat the coronectomy in cases of failure. J Oral Maxillofac Surg. 2015;73:587–94. https://doi.org/10.1016/j.joms.2014.10.011.
18. Abu-Mostafa N, AlRejaie LM, Almutairi FA, Alajaji RA, Alkodair MM, Alzahem NA. Evaluation of the outcomes of coronectomy procedure versus surgical extraction of lower third molars which have a high risk for inferior alveolar nerve injury: a systematic review. Int J Dent. 2021;2021:9161606. https://doi.org/10.1155/2021/9161606.
19. Lee NJ, Jung SY, Park KM, Choi Y, Huh J, Park W. Factors affecting root migration after coronectomy of the mandibular third molar. Medicine. 2021;100:e25974. https://doi.org/10.1097/MD.0000000000025974.
20. Monaco G, Angelino C, Vignudelli E, Ferri A, Felice P. What is the incidence of late complications associated with lower third molar coronectomy? 10-year follow-up results. J Oral Maxillofac Surg. 2023;81:1279–85. https://doi.org/10.1016/j.joms.2023.06.011.
21. Hamad SA. Outcomes of coronectomy and total odontectomy of impacted mandibular third molars. Int Dent J. 2024;74(2):195–8. https://doi.org/10.1016/j.identj.2023.07.015.
22. Pitros P, O'Connor N, Tryfonos A, Lopes V. A systematic review of the complications of high-risk third molar removal and coronectomy: development of a decision tree model and preliminary health economic analysis to assist in treatment planning. Br J Oral Maxillofac Surg. 2020;58:e16–24. https://doi.org/10.1016/j.bjoms.2020.07.015.
23. Nishimoto RN, Moshman AT, Dodson TB, Beirne OR. Why is mandibular third molar coronectomy successful without concurrent root canal treatment? J Oral Maxillofac Surg. 2020;78:1886–91. https://doi.org/10.1016/j.joms.2020.05.046.
24. Fraser J. No coronectomy. Br Dent J. 2020;228:227. https://doi.org/10.1038/s41415-020-1321-4.
25. Bonetti GA, Parenti SI, Checchi L. Orthodontic extraction of mandibular third molar to avoid nerve injury and promote periodontal healing. J Clin Periodontol. 2008;35:719–23. https://doi.org/10.1111/j.1600-051X.2008.01286.x.
26. Hirsch A, Shteiman S, Boyan BD, Schwartz Z. Use of orthodontic treatment as an aid to third molar extraction: a method for prevention of mandibular nerve injury and improved periodontal status. J Periodontol. 2003;74:887–92. https://doi.org/10.1902/jop.2003.74.6.887.
27. Kalantar Motamedi MR, Heidarpour M, Siadat S, Kalantar Motamedi A, Bahreman AA. Orthodontic extraction of high-risk impacted mandibular third molars in close proximity to the mandibular canal: a systematic review. J Oral Maxillofac Surg. 2015;73:1672–85. https://doi.org/10.1016/j.joms.2015.03.031.
28. Wang Z, Liu Z, Shi Y, Fang D, Li S, Zhang D. A novel orthodontic extraction method for removal of impacted mandibular third molars in close proximity to inferior alveolar nerve. J Oral Maxillofac Surg. 2019;77:1575.e1–6. https://doi.org/10.1016/j.joms.2019.04.013.
29. Jung S, Lee JH, Huh J, Park W. Orthodontic extrusion of mandibular third molar with a miniscrew and cross-arch elastic. J Oral Maxillofac Surg. 2021;79:1422.e1–8. https://doi.org/10.1016/j.joms.2021.01.036.
30. Grassi A, Monica D, Minetti E, et al. Innovative alveolar ridge preservation surgical technique with immediate dental implant placement: a retrospective case report of 1-year follow-up. Eur J Dent. 2024;18(1):408–14. https://doi.org/10.1055/s-0043-1772676.
31. You S, Yu F, Fan Q, et al. Radiographic comparison of atelocollagen versus deproteinized bovine bone minerals covered with a collagen membrane in alveolar ridge preservation: a retrospective study. BMC Oral Health. 2023;23:901. https://doi.org/10.1186/s12903-023-03647-y.
32. Quisiguiña Salem C, Ruiz Delgado E, Crespo Reinoso PA, Robalino JJ. Alveolar ridge preservation: a review of concepts and controversies. Natl J Maxillofac Surg. 2023;14:167–76. https://doi.org/10.4103/njms.njms_224_22.
33. Stumbras A, Kuliesius P, Januzis G, Juodzbalys G. Alveolar ridge preservation after tooth extrac-

tion using different bone graft materials and autologous platelet concentrates: a systematic review. J Oral Maxillofac Res. 2019;10(1):e2. https://doi.org/10.5037/jomr.2019.10102.

34. Bavetta G, Licata ME. The use of human allogenic graft (HBA) for maxillary bone regeneration: review of literature and case reports. Curr Pharm Des. 2012;18:5559–68. https://doi.org/10.2174/138161212803307572.
35. Khan RS, Aslam M, Ucer C, Wright S. Success of xenografts in alveolar ridge preservation based on histomorphometric outcomes. Dent J. 2023;11:215. https://doi.org/10.3390/dj11090215.
36. Majzoub J, Ravida A, Starch-Jensen T, Tattan M, Suárez-López Del Amo F. The influence of different grafting materials on alveolar ridge preservation: a systematic review. J Oral Maxillofac Res. 2019;10:e6. https://doi.org/10.5037/jomr.2019.10306.
37. Kormas I, Pedercini A, Alassy H, Wolff LF. The use of biocompatible membranes in oral surgery: the past, present & future directions. A narrative review. Membranes. 2022;12:841. https://doi.org/10.3390/membranes12090841.
38. Steigmann L, Di Gianfilippo R, Steigmann M, Wang HL. Classification based on extraction socket buccal bone morphology and related treatment decision tree. Materials. 2022;15:733. https://doi.org/10.3390/ma1503073.
39. Del Fabbro M, Tommasato G, Pesce P, et al. Sealing materials for post-extraction site: a systematic review and network meta-analysis. Clin Oral Investig. 2022;26:1137–54. https://doi.org/10.1007/s00784-021-04262-3.
40. Lim HC, Shin HS, Cho IW, Koo KT, Park JC. Ridge preservation in molar extraction sites with an open-healing approach: a randomized controlled clinical trial. J Clin Periodontol. 2019;46:1144–54.
41. Lekovic V, Camargo PM, Klokkevold PR, et al. Preservation of alveolar bone in extraction sockets using bioabsorbable membranes. J Periodontol. 1998;69:1044–9.
42. Elayah SA, Younis H, Cui H, et al. Alveolar ridge preservation in post-extraction sockets using concentrated growth factors: a split-mouth, randomized, controlled clinical trial. Front Endocrinol. 2023;14:1163696. https://doi.org/10.3389/fendo.2023.1163696.
43. Morris ML. The implantation of decalcified human dentin and cementum into the subcutaneous tissues of the rat. J Periodontal Res. 1967;2:273–81. https://doi.org/10.1111/j.1600-0765.1967.tb01899.x.
44. Morris ML. The implantation of decalcified human dentin and cementum with autogenous bone and marrow into the subcutaneous tissues of the rat. J Periodontol. 1969;40:731–5. https://doi.org/10.1902/jop.1969.40.12.731.
45. Morris ML. The implantation of human dentin and cementum with autogenous red marrow into the subcutaneous tissues of the rat. J Periodontol. 1969;40:571–6. https://doi.org/10.1902/jop.1969.40.10.571.
46. Morris ML. The implantation of human dentin and cementum with autogenous bone and red marrow into the subcutaneous tissues of the rat. J Periodontol. 1969;40:259–63. https://doi.org/10.1902/jop.1969.40.5.259.
47. Jeong K-I, Kim S-G, Kim Y-K, Oh J-S, Jeong M-A, Park J-J. Clinical study of graft materials using autogenous teeth in maxillary sinus augmentation. Implant Dent. 2011;20:471–5. https://doi.org/10.1097/ID.0b013e3182386d74.
48. Pang KM, Um IW, Kim YK, Woo JM, Kim SM, Lee JH. Autogenous demineralized dentin matrix from extracted tooth for the augmentation of alveolar bone defect: a prospective randomized clinical trial in comparison with anorganic bovine bone. Clin Oral Implants Res. 2017;28:809–15. https://doi.org/10.1111/clr.12885.
49. Joshi CP, Dani NH, Khedkar SU. Alveolar ridge preservation using autogenous tooth graft versus beta-tricalcium phosphate alloplast: a randomized, controlled, prospective, clinical pilot study. J Indian Soc Periodontol. 2016;20:429–34. https://doi.org/10.4103/0972-124X.188335.
50. Park SM, Um IW, Kim YK, Kim KW. Clinical application of autotooth bone graft material. J Korean Assoc Oral Maxillofac Surg. 2012;38:2–8.
51. Hashemi S, Tabatabaei S, Fathi A, Asadinejad SM, Atash R. Tooth graft: an umbrella overview. Eur J Dent. 2024;18(1):41–54. https://doi.org/10.1055/s-0043-1764420.
52. Sánchez-Labrador L, Bazal-Bonelli S, Pérez-González F, Sáez-Alcaide LM, Cortés-Bretón Brinkmann J, Martínez-González JM. Autogenous particulated dentin for alveolar ridge preservation. A systematic review. Ann Anat. 2023;246:152024. https://doi.org/10.1016/j.aanat.2022.152024.
53. Lee EY, Kim ES, Kim KW. Scanning electron microscopy and energy dispersive x-ray spectroscopy studies on processed tooth graft material by vacuum-ultrasonic acceleration. Maxillofac Plast Reconstr Surg. 2014;36:103–10. https://doi.org/10.14402/jkamprs.2014.36.3.103.
54. Kim KW. Bone induction by demineralized dentin matrix in nude mouse muscles. Maxillofac Plast Reconstr Surg. 2014;36:50–6. https://doi.org/10.14402/jkamprs.2014.36.2.50.
55. Santos A, Botelho J, Machado V, et al. Autogenous mineralized dentin versus xenograft granules in ridge preservation for delayed implantation in post-extraction sites: a randomized controlled clinical trial with an 18 months follow-up. Clin Oral Implants Res. 2021;32:905–15. https://doi.org/10.1111/clr.13765.
56. Vaia E, Nicolò M, Vaia E, Iorio-Siciliano V, Isola G, Ramaglia L. Alveolar ridge preservation with deproteinized bovine bone mineral and xenogeneic collagen matrix: a 12-month clinical and histomorphometric case series. Int J Periodontics Restorative Dent. 2021;41:423–30. https://doi.org/10.11607/prd.4606.
57. Iasella JM, Greenwell H, Miller RL, et al. Ridge preservation with freeze-dried bone allograft and a

collagen membrane compared to extraction alone for implant site development: a clinical and histologic study in humans. J Periodontol. 2003;74:990–9. https://doi.org/10.1902/jop.2003.74.7.990.
58. Girish Kumar N, Chaudhary R, Kumar I, Arora SS, Kumar N, Singh H. To assess the efficacy of socket plug technique using platelet rich fibrin with or without the use of bone substitute in alveolar ridge preservation: a prospective randomised controlled study. Oral Maxillofac Surg. 2018;22:135–42. https://doi.org/10.1007/s10006-018-0680-3.
59. Yalcin S, Aktas I, Emes Y, Kaya G, Aybar B, Atalay B. A technique for atraumatic extraction of teeth before immediate implant placement using implant drills. Implant Dent. 2009;18:464–72. https://doi.org/10.1097/ID.0b013e3181bcc6d9.
60. Demirci A, Bayram F, Dergin G. Piezosurgery versus conventional rotary surgery for impacted third molars: a randomised, split-mouth, clinical pilot trial. Med Oral Patol Oral Cir Bucal. 2024;29(1):e1–8. https://doi.org/10.4317/medoral.25929.
61. Mahardawi B, Jiaranuchart S, Arunjaroensuk S, Tompkins KA, Somboonsavatdee A, Pimkhaokham A. The effect of different hemostatic agents following dental extraction in patients under oral antithrombotic therapy: a network meta-analysis. Sci Rep. 2023;13:12519. https://doi.org/10.1038/s41598-023-39023-7.
62. Guo Y, Wang M, Liu Q, Liu G, Wang S, Li J. Recent advances in the medical applications of hemostatic materials. Theranostics. 2023;13:161–96. https://doi.org/10.7150/thno.79639.

MIX
Papier aus verantwortungsvollen Quellen
Paper from responsible sources
FSC® C105338

If you have any concerns about our products,
you can contact us on
**ProductSafety@springernature.com**

In case Publisher is established outside the EU,
the EU authorized representative is:
**Springer Nature Customer Service Center GmbH**
**Europaplatz 3, 69115 Heidelberg, Germany**

Printed by Libri Plureos GmbH
in Hamburg, Germany